PUBLIC HEALTH IN THE 21ST CENTURY

FEDERAL PROGRAMS SUPPORTING PEOPLE WITH SERIOUS MENTAL ILLNESS

AN ASSESSMENT

PUBLIC HEALTH IN THE 21ST CENTURY

Additional books in this series can be found on Nova's website under the Series tab.

Additional e-books in this series can be found on Nova's website under the e-book tab.

PUBLIC HEALTH IN THE 21ST CENTURY

FEDERAL PROGRAMS SUPPORTING PEOPLE WITH SERIOUS MENTAL ILLNESS

AN ASSESSMENT

BENJAMIN WRIGHT
EDITOR

NOVINKA

New York

Library of Congress Cataloging-in-Publication Data

ISBN: 978-1-63483-043-0

Published by Nova Science Publishers, Inc. † New York

CONTENTS

PREFACE

In 2013, about 10 million adults in the United States had a serious mental illness. The U.S. mental health care system includes a range of federal programs—across multiple agencies—for those with mental illness. Past efforts to develop a list of federal programs supporting individuals with serious mental illness have highlighted the difficulty of identifying such programs. This book identifies the federal programs that support individuals with serious mental illness; the extent to which federal agencies coordinate these programs; and the extent to which federal agencies evaluate such programs.

Determining how many people have a mental illness can be difficult, and prevalence estimates vary. While numerous surveys include questions related to mental illness, few provide prevalence estimates of diagnosable mental illness (e.g., major depressive disorder as opposed to feeling depressed, or generalized anxiety disorder as opposed to feeling anxious), and fewer still provide national prevalence estimates of diagnosable mental illness. This book briefly describes the methodology and results of three large surveys that provide national prevalence estimates of diagnosable mental illness.

In: Federal Programs
Editor: Benjamin Wright

ISBN: 978-1-63483-043-0

Chapter 1

MENTAL HEALTH: HHS LEADERSHIP NEEDED TO COORDINATE FEDERAL EFFORTS RELATED TO SERIOUS MENTAL ILLNESS*

United States Government Accountability Office

WHY GAO DID THIS STUDY

In 2013, about 10 million adults in the United States had a serious mental illness. The U.S. mental health care system includes a range of federal programs—across multiple agencies—for those with mental illness. Past efforts to develop a list of federal programs supporting individuals with serious mental illness have highlighted the difficulty of identifying such programs.

GAO was asked to provide information on federal programs that support individuals with serious mental illness. This report identifies (1) the federal programs that support individuals with serious mental illness; (2) the extent to which federal agencies coordinate these programs; and (3) the extent to which federal agencies evaluate such programs. GAO developed and administered a web-based questionnaire to eight federal agencies regarding program goals,

* This is an edited, reformatted and augmented version of a United States Government Accountability Office publication, No. GAO-15-113, dated December 2014.

target populations, services offered, evaluations, and coordination. GAO also interviewed agency officials.

What GAO Recommends

GAO recommends that HHS establish a mechanism to facilitate interagency coordination across programs that support individuals with serious mental illness. GAO also recommends that DOD, HHS, DOJ, and VA document which programs targeting individuals with serious mental illness should be evaluated and how often such evaluations should be completed. HHS disagreed with both recommendations. DOD, DOJ, and VA agreed with the second recommendation. GAO continues to believe the recommendations are valid as discussed in the report.

What GAO Found

Agencies identified 112 federal programs that generally supported individuals with serious mental illness in fiscal year 2013. The majority of these programs addressed broad issues, such as homelessness, that can include individuals with serious mental illness. The programs were spread across eight federal agencies: Department of Defense (DOD), Department of Education, Department of Health and Human Services (HHS), Department of Housing and Urban Development, Department of Justice (DOJ), Department of Labor, Department of Veterans Affairs (VA), and the Social Security Administration. Thirty of the 112 programs were identified by the agencies as specifically targeting individuals with serious mental illness. Four agencies—DOD, HHS, DOJ, and VA—reported that they obligated about $5.7 billion for programs that specifically targeted individuals with serious mental illness in fiscal year 2013. Agencies had difficulty identifying all programs supporting individuals with serious mental illness because they did not always track whether or not such individuals were among those served by the program. Agencies also varied in which programs they identified because they had different definitions of what such a program might be. Such inconsistency limits the potential comparability across programs.

Interagency coordination for programs supporting individuals with serious mental illness is lacking. HHS is charged with leading the federal government's public health efforts related to mental health, and the Substance Abuse and Mental Health Services Administration is required to promote coordination of programs relating to mental illness throughout the federal government. In the past, HHS led the Federal Executive Steering Committee for Mental Health, with members from across the federal government. However, the steering committee has not met since 2009. HHS officials told us that the Behavioral Health Coordinating Council (BHCC) performs some functions previously carried out by the steering committee. The BHCC, however, is limited to HHS and is not an interagency committee. Other interagency committees were broad in scope and did not target individuals with serious mental illness. Staff for the majority of the programs targeting serious mental illness reported taking steps to coordinate with staff in other agencies. While coordination at the program level is important, it does not take the place of, or achieve the level of, leadership that GAO has previously found to be key to successful coordination and that is essential to identifying whether there are gaps in services and if agencies have the necessary information to assess the reach and effectiveness of their programs.

Agencies completed few evaluations of the programs specifically targeting individuals with serious mental illness. Of the 30 programs specifically targeting individuals with serious mental illness, 9 programs had a completed program evaluation, 4 programs had an evaluation underway, and 17 programs had no evaluation completed and none planned. However, agency officials said they engaged in other efforts—such as drawing on evidence in published literature— to ensure their programs were effective. GAO's prior work has shown the significance of both performance monitoring activities and program evaluations and noted the importance of formal program evaluations to inform program managers about the overall design and operation of the program.

ABBREVIATIONS

BHCC	Behavioral Health Coordinating Council
DOD	Department of Defense
DOJ	Department of Justice
DOL	Department of Labor
DSM	Diagnostic and Statistical Manual of Mental Disorders
Education	Department of Education
GPRA	Government Performance and Results Act of 1993
HHS	Department of Health and Human Services

HUD	Department of Housing and Urban Development
OMB	Office of Management and Budget
PAIMI	Protection and Advocacy for Individuals with Mental Illness
PTSD	post-traumatic stress disorder
SAMHSA	Substance Abuse and Mental Health Services Administration
SSA	Social Security Administration
VA	Department of Veterans Affairs

* * *

December 18, 2014

The Honorable Tim Murphy
Chairman
The Honorable Diana DeGette
Ranking Member
Subcommittee on Oversight and Investigations
Committee on Energy and Commerce
House of Representatives

Mental illness is widespread in the United States. According to figures from the Substance Abuse and Mental Health Services Administration (SAMHSA)—an agency within the Department of Health and Human Services (HHS)—an estimated 43.8 million—or 18.5 percent—of adults in the United States suffered from a mental illness in 2013.[1] Among those, about 10 million—or 4.2 percent—of adults in the United States suffered from a serious mental illness, which generally includes conditions such as schizophrenia, bipolar disorder, major depression, and severe post-traumatic stress disorder (PTSD).[2] Children also suffer from mental health issues. In 2013, approximately 10.7 percent of children—an estimated 2.6 million—aged 12 to 17 years old experienced a period of major depression.[3]

The U.S. mental health care system includes a range of programs for those with a mental illness, including programs addressing broad social issues, such as homelessness, that can generally support individuals with mental illness as well as other programs that are specifically targeting people with mental illness. The federal government provides a range of programs to support the needs of individuals with serious mental illness. There have been efforts in the past to develop a list of the federal programs and resources that are devoted to supporting and treating individuals with serious mental illness, and some have highlighted the difficulty of identifying all of the programs. For example, in 2013, the Office of Management and Budget (OMB) collected information on the federal activities and services that support individuals with mental illness; however, OMB acknowledged that the information gathered did not include a number of federal programs that address mental health as part of broader activities and that there are also services or benefits provided to individuals with mental illness that are not provided exclusively on the basis of an individual's mental illness.[4]

Because of the size of the population affected and the complexity of treating those with mental illness, coordinating and evaluating programs that support these individuals is particularly important for meeting the needs of this vulnerable population. Both Congress and the executive branch have recognized the need for improved collaboration across the federal government, and many of the meaningful results that the federal government seeks to achieve require the coordinated efforts of government agencies. Our prior work has highlighted some of the approaches and key considerations for implementing interagency collaborative mechanisms, such as defining outcomes; measuring performance and ensuring accountability; and establishing leadership approaches, among other things.[5] Furthermore, evaluation can play a key role in agency strategic planning and in program management, providing important feedback on both program design and execution.

You asked us to provide information on how federal agencies support programs for individuals with serious mental illness and ensure these programs are meeting the needs of this population. This report identifies (1) the federal programs that support individuals with serious mental illness; (2) the extent to which federal agencies coordinate programs for individuals with serious mental illness; and (3) the extent to which federal agencies evaluate or monitor programs for individuals with serious mental illness.

To identify federal programs supporting those with serious mental illness, the extent to which federal agencies are coordinating, and the extent to which federal agencies evaluate or monitor programs, we developed a web-based questionnaire.[6] The web-based questionnaire asked questions about program goals, target populations, services offered, performance information and evaluations, coordination, and funding in fiscal year 2013. To determine which federal departments, agencies, and other federal entities administer programs that support individuals with serious mental illness, we reviewed existing documentation and reports and interviewed advocacy groups and agency officials.[7] Based on this review and our interviews, we identified eight agencies frequently cited as having relevant programs supporting individuals with serious mental illness and administered the questionnaire to those agencies.[8] We supplemented the questionnaire responses with follow-up interviews and questions to each of the agencies to obtain any additional information. To assess the reliability of the information we received, we performed internal reliability checks and conducted follow-up as necessary with agency officials. As a result, we determined that the data used in our report were sufficiently reliable for our purposes. See appendix I for more information on our scope and methodology.

We conducted this performance audit from December 2013 to December 2014 in accordance with generally accepted government auditing standards. Those standards require that we plan and perform the audit to obtain sufficient, appropriate evidence to provide a reasonable basis for our findings and conclusions based on our audit objectives. We believe that the evidence obtained provides a reasonable basis for our findings and conclusions based on our audit objectives.

BACKGROUND

Mental Illness

Mental illness is generally defined as a health condition that changes a person's thinking, feelings, or behavior and causes the person distress and difficulty in functioning.[9] The symptoms associated with a given type of mental illness can vary in frequency and severity across individuals and for each individual over time. Mental illnesses with particularly severe symptoms can have a dramatic impact on an individual's ability to function in everyday life. The fatigue experienced by an individual with major depressive disorder can be so severe that it is difficult to summon the energy to work every day. The delusions associated with paranoid schizophrenia can make it impossible to maintain stable personal relationships with spouses, co-workers, or friends. Certain other mental illnesses are known for the unpredictable and episodic nature of their symptoms and the harmful effect this has on the ability to function consistently over time. For example, individuals with bipolar disorder can alternate between periods of mania, relative normalcy, and profound depression.

Mental Health Care System

The services provided by the public mental health care system to individuals with serious mental illness have changed over time. Historically, state-run public mental health hospitals were the principal treatment option available to them. By the 1960s, the reliance on inpatient care was viewed as ineffective and inadequate because of patient overcrowding, staff shortages, and other factors. At the same time, improved medications and other interventions were reducing some of the symptoms of mental illness and increasing the potential for more of these individuals to live successfully in the community. A recovery-oriented, community-based approach to mental health treatment has since emerged. Under this approach, individuals are to receive services and supports uniquely designed to help them manage their mental illness and to maximize their potential to live independently in the community. These services and supports are multidimensional—intended to address not only mental illness but also employment, housing, and other issues. When feasible, these multidimensional services are provided in what is referred to as a "wrap-around" manner—that is, they are uniquely targeted to the nature and extent of each individual's needs. When services are provided by multiple agencies, those agencies are to coordinate their activities and funding so that the individual experiences the services and supports seamlessly—as if from one system, not many.

Federal Mental Health Care Programs

The federal government provides a range of programs to support the needs of individuals with serious mental illness, such as funding block grants to community mental health organizations and providing supportive housing programs for individuals with mental illness. The responsibility for the administration and evaluation of these programs falls upon multiple agencies, including Department of Defense (DOD), Department of Education (Education), HHS, Department of Housing and Urban Development (HUD), Department of Justice (DOJ), Department of Labor (DOL), Department of Veterans Affairs (VA), and Social Security Administration (SSA). Programs supporting individuals with serious mental illness may or may not be specifically targeting that population. For example, a program providing housing for homeless veterans may provide support to individuals with serious mental illness because these individuals make up a portion of the population of homeless veterans, but the program is targeting homeless veterans rather than individuals with serious mental illness.

SAMHSA, an agency within HHS, leads the federal government's public health efforts related to behavioral health, which includes mental health.[10] Specifically, SAMHSA administers behavioral health programs, disseminates policies, information and data, and awards contracts and grants to states, tribes, local governments, and other organizations, including those that support individuals with serious mental illness.[11]

Agency Coordination and Program Evaluation

Our prior work has noted the importance of coordinating and evaluating programs. This is particularly important in the case of federal efforts to support serious mental illness, given the size of the population affected and the complexity of treatment. We have also reported on the importance of coordination between federal agencies on issues of national significance as a way to avoid fragmentation.[12] Many of the meaningful results that the federal government seeks to achieve require the coordinated efforts of more than one federal agency and often more than one sector and level of government. Our past work has identified a range of mechanisms that the federal government uses to lead and implement interagency coordination, including interagency groups sometimes referred to as task forces, working groups, councils, or committees.[13]

In addition, for many years, we have reported that more frequent evaluations of performance and results were needed for multiple federal programs and activities.[14] A program evaluation is an individual, systematic study to assess how well a program or programs are working.

Evaluations answer specific questions about program performance and may focus on assessing program operations or results. Evaluation can play a key role in agency strategic planning and in program management, providing important feedback on both program design and execution.[15] Program evaluation is closely related to performance measurement and reporting. Performance measurement is the systematic ongoing monitoring and reporting of program accomplishments, particularly progress toward established goals or standards. The Government Performance and Results Act of 1993 (GPRA), as expanded by the GPRA Modernization Act of 2010, encourages federal agencies to conduct evaluations by requiring them to include a schedule of future program evaluations in their strategic plans and summarize their evaluation findings when reporting on their performance goals, among other things.[16]

EIGHT AGENCIES REPORTED OVER 100 PROGRAMS THAT CAN SUPPORT INDIVIDUALS WITH SERIOUS MENTAL ILLNESS, BUT IT IS UNLIKELY ALL PROGRAMS WERE IDENTIFIED

Agencies Identified 112 Programs That Can Support Individuals with Serious Mental Illness, 30 of Which Specifically Target This Population

Agencies identified 112 federal programs in fiscal year 2013—across eight federal agencies—that can support individuals with serious mental illness. These 112 programs conducted activities that can generally support individuals with serious mental illness. For example, HUD's Continuum of Care program provided funding to nonprofit providers and state and local governments to quickly find housing for homeless individuals and families, among other services. See appendix II for a list of the 112 federal programs identified as supporting individuals with serious mental illness in fiscal year 2013.[17]

The number and purpose of programs identified by agencies through our questionnaire varied widely. [18] DOD reported the largest number, a total of 34 programs, and HHS identified 33. Together, the agencies accounted for more than half of the 112 programs.[19] DOJ and VA also each reported over 10 programs. Overall, many of the programs focused on the provision of support services and a few programs focused on research or surveillance. Programs that provided support services included those that provided case management services such as SAMHSA's Criminal and Juvenile Justice Programs. These programs sought to divert individuals with serious mental illness from the criminal justice system by providing support services that connect the individual to behavioral health, housing, and job placement services. DOD was the only agency that reported prevention programs (13 programs) through the questionnaire, and three agencies—DOD, HHS, and VA—reported treatment programs (16 programs). About a quarter of the programs—27 programs—were identified as serving other purposes. For example, the Department of Education included its Personnel Development program that awarded grants to assist in ensuring adequate numbers of highly qualified special education teachers and fully certified personnel to serve children with disabilities, including children with serious emotional disturbance who may have a serious mental illness. Table 1 provides the number of these programs, by primary program purpose, within the eight federal agencies.

Table 1. Programs That Can Support Individuals with Serious Mental Illness Identified by Eight Federal Agencies in Fiscal Year 2013, by Primary Program Purpose

	Number of programs, by primary program purpose								
Agency	Prevention	Research	Support services	Surveillance	Technical assistance	Treatment	Other	Not identified	Total
DOD	13		11	1		4	5		34
DOJ			7				4		11
DOL			1		1		6		8
Education		1			1		5		7
HHS		1	13		3	3	1	12	33
HUD							4[a]		4
SSA		1	2				1		4
VA			1			9	1		11
Total	13	3	35	1	5	16	27	12[b]	112

Source: GAO analysis of questionnaire responses and interviews with eight federal agencies. | GAO-15-113

Legend:

DOD	Department of Defense
DOJ	Department of Justice
DOL	Department of Labor
Education	Department of Education
HHS	Department of Health and Human Services
HUD	Department of Housing and Urban Development
SSA	Social Security Administration
VA	Department of Veterans Affairs

Note: The scope of this report did not include health benefit programs—such as Medicaid, Medicare, and TRICARE—that reimburse providers for various mental health services.

[a]HUD submitted five programs with the primary purpose "other." One of the programs, HUD-VA Supportive Housing, was also submitted by VA. To avoid double-counting we included this program under VA.

[b]In addition to completing the questionnaire for 13 programs they administer that are targeted to individuals with serious mental illness, Substance Abuse and Mental Health Services Administration (SAMHSA) officials also provided the names of 12 programs that can offer general support to individuals with serious mental illness. SAMHSA officials did not identify the primary purpose for these programs.

In addition to serving a variety of purposes the 112 programs that support individuals with serious mental illness, served a variety of subpopulations, ranging from children to homeless veterans. For example, DOJ administered a program—the Second Chance Act Reentry Program—that focused on adults and youth with co-occurring substance abuse and mental health disorders during their confinement or court supervision. In addition, DOL administered the Homeless Veterans Reintegration program, which worked to meet the needs of homeless veterans by reintegrating them into the workforce.

A subset of the 112 programs—30 programs, or 27 percent—were identified by agencies as specifically targeting individuals with serious mental illness.[20] These targeted programs were administered by five agencies: DOD, DOJ, HHS, SSA, and VA. The primary purpose of the 30 targeted programs varied. Half of the targeted programs (15 programs) provided support services, such as case management, to individuals with serious mental illness. Ten of those programs were within HHS. Seven of the targeted programs provided treatment services, with 6 of those programs—administered by VA—providing treatment services to veterans with serious mental illness. All targeted programs reported by HHS were within SAMHSA, and focused on providing support services and technical assistance.[21] Table 2 provides the number of these programs, by primary program purpose, within the five federal agencies that identified programs specifically targeted towards individuals with serious mental illness.

In addition to serving a variety of purposes, the 30 programs that specifically target individuals with serious mental illness, served a variety of subpopulations, ranging from children and families to homeless veterans. Over half of the targeted programs (16 programs) were administered by three agencies—DOD, DOJ, and VA—and served specific subpopulations; servicemembers, incarcerated or previously incarcerated individuals, and veterans, respectively. Three of the targeted programs (all within HHS) served children and/or families. The remaining programs served adults.

Table 2. Programs That Specifically Target Individuals with Serious Mental Illness Administered by Eight Federal Agencies in Fiscal Year 2013, by Primary Program Purpose

	Number of programs, by primary program purpose							
Agency	Prevention	Research	Support services	Surveillance	Technical assistance	Treatment	Other	Total
DOD	3		1			1		5
DOJ			3					3
HHS			10		3			13
SSA		1						1
VA			1			6	1	8
Total	3	1	15		3	7	1	30

Source: GAO analysis of questionnaire responses from five federal agencies. | GAO-15-113

Legend:

DOD Department of Defense

DOJ Department of Justice

HHS Department of Health and Human Services

SSA Social Security Administration

VA Department of Veterans Affairs

Based on agency-reported information from the questionnaire, about $5.7 billion was obligated for the 30 targeted programs in fiscal year 2013.[22] The majority of these funds—84 percent—was obligated by DOD and VA for treatment and support services (among other things) for servicemembers, veterans and their families.[23] HHS's SAMHSA obligations represented about 13 percent of total obligations for the 30 targeted programs.[24] HHS officials noted that Medicaid is the largest payer for services for individuals with serious mental illness and that Medicare is also a significant payer for services for that population.[25] The remaining funds were obligated for programs within DOJ.[26] See appendix III for more information on the 30 targeted programs.

It Is Unlikely That Agencies Identified All Programs for Individuals with Serious Mental Illness

Agencies had difficulty identifying all programs supporting individuals with serious mental illness because they did not always track whether or not such individuals were among the population served by the program. During follow-up interviews, officials from several agencies indicated that they were unsure how many individuals with serious mental illness were served by various programs. Specifically, some agencies noted that they administered broad federal programs focusing on individuals with disabilities that could serve individuals with serious mental illness. For example, Education officials indicated that individuals with serious mental illness could have been among individuals eligible to receive services under their Centers for Independent Living program that provided financial assistance to community-based centers for independent living.[27]

However, Education officials were unsure the extent to which the program served individuals with serious mental illness because that was not the focus of the program and because individuals self-identify their disability, which may include a serious mental illness. Similarly, the Disability Employment Initiative administered by DOL served all people with disabilities, including individuals with serious mental illness, but it was unclear how many individuals with serious mental illness were served by this program. Officials from agencies within HHS also noted that it is possible that all of their programs could support individuals with serious mental illness.

The inability of agencies to identify a comprehensive list or inventory of programs for individuals with serious mental illness is problematic. The GPRA Modernization Act of 2010 requires OMB to compile a comprehensive list of all federal programs identified by agencies, and to include the purposes of each program, how it contributes to the agency's mission, and recent funding information.[28] However, as we reported earlier this year, our initial review of these lists identified concerns about the usefulness of the information being developed and the extent to which it might be able to assist executive branch and congressional efforts to identify and address fragmentation, overlap, and duplication.[29] The lack of such a list makes it more difficult for executive branch agencies and Congress to determine whether proposed or existing programs are duplicative.

In addition to difficulties in identifying a comprehensive inventory of programs for individuals with serious mental illness, some agencies also had difficulty identifying how much funding was obligated for programs supporting individuals with serious mental illness. For example, HHS's National Institutes of Health identified all of its activities, including its mental health activities as one program, Scientific Research. Officials said they were able to identify funding amounts for individual research studies related to certain illnesses that may be considered serious mental illnesses, such as depression or schizophrenia. 30 They noted that they were currently developing a method to categorize all research grants that were related to serious mental illness. Similarly, DOJ's Bureau of Prisons identified three programs targeting individuals with serious mental illness but could not provide the obligated funding amounts for the programs, providing instead an amount that included all psychology services programs, which included all of the Bureau of Prisons' substance abuse and mental health programs.

In addition, the number and scope of programs agencies identified is likely incomplete and difficult to compare across agencies for a variety of other reasons. Agencies varied widely in how they counted their programs, resulting in inconsistencies among agencies, thus limiting the potential comparability across programs.[31] Some agencies identified broad programs that included many activities; other agencies counted each of these underlying activities as a separate program. For example, within DOD, the Army included one program, the Behavioral Health System of Care, which included a broad array of mental health and substance abuse activities for servicemembers and their families. In contrast, the Navy chose to list each comparable behavioral health activity as a separate program. Furthermore, NIH identified only one program, its Scientific Research program, which encompassed all of its internal and external research project grants on topics ranging from cardiovascular health to those grants related to mental illness.[32]

Agencies also varied in how they defined their programs and in which programs they chose to include.[33] For example, DOD officials identified all of their suicide prevention programs as those that support individuals with serious mental illness, but SAMHSA officials did not initially include any of their suicide prevention programs. They explained that these services were not limited only to individuals with serious mental illness and served a broader population. Subsequently, after further discussion with us, SAMHSA included their suicide prevention programs among those that can support individuals with serious mental illness. In another instance, HUD and VA jointly administered the HUD-VA Supportive Housing program, a specialized program aimed at providing housing and other services to disabled veterans. VA officials indicated that this program was targeting individuals with serious mental illness while HUD maintained that the program was not targeting this population. Similar to these challenges in identifying programs supporting individuals with serious mental illness, our prior work has also found that agencies took various approaches to defining their programs. This variation in definitions across agencies can limit comparability among similar programs.[34]

INTERAGENCY COORDINATION OF PROGRAMS SUPPORTING PEOPLE WITH SERIOUS MENTAL ILLNESS IS LACKING

Agency-level committees that officials said allowed them to coordinate efforts regarding mental health did not focus on, and took little action specific to, serious mental illness. However, program staff for the majority of the programs targeting serious mental illness reported taking steps to coordinate with other program-level staff.

Committees Have Been Established for Interagency Coordination, but They Did Not Focus on, and Took Little Action Specific to, Serious Mental Illness

Interagency coordination for programs for individuals with serious mental illness is lacking because agency-level committees do not focus specifically on, and have taken little action regarding, serious mental illness. While DOD, DOJ, HHS, SSA, and VA officials reported establishing committees that they said allow them to coordinate efforts regarding mental health across agencies, none of these committees were focused specifically on serious mental illness.[35] In 2003, the President's New Freedom Commission on Mental Health produced a report on the fragmentation among programs for individuals with serious mental illness and made recommendations to the federal government to better coordinate services. In response, the Federal Executive Steering Committee for Mental Health—led by HHS—was formed with high-level representatives from DOD, DOJ, DOL, Education, HUD, SSA, VA, the Department of Agriculture, and the Department of Transportation. In 2008, we reported that the committee had taken steps to coordinate federal efforts by promoting access to employment services for young adults with serious mental illness.[36] However, the steering committee has not met since 2009. HHS officials told us that the Behavioral Health Coordinating Council (BHCC) performs some functions previously carried out by the steering committee. The Secretary of HHS established the BHCC in 2010 to bring together members from agencies within HHS to focus on behavioral health issues, but the council did not include officials from other federal agencies. Moreover, the BHCC has focused mainly on substance use issues, rather than mental health.[37]

There are several other interagency committees according to agency officials, but these committees were generally broader in scope and did not specifically focus on individuals with serious mental illness. (See table 3 for several examples of such committees that are currently operational.) For example, DOD, HHS, and VA lead the Interagency Task Force on Military and Veterans Mental Health to provide support to veterans, servicemembers, and their families.[38] Agency officials told us the Interagency Task Force has undertaken efforts that were broadly related to mental health such as expanding capacity for mental health treatment, but have taken few actions specifically targeting serious mental illness. Similarly, HHS officials reported that the U.S. Interagency Council on Homelessness—formed to coordinate the federal response to homelessness—has worked to improve access to behavioral health services in an effort to address chronic and veteran homelessness.

Accordingly, the work of this committee might affect individuals with serious mental illness, but the committee did not specifically focus on the unique needs of this population. Only one of the identified committees—HHS's BHCC—had plans to establish a subcommittee devoted to addressing serious mental illness. It is also important to note that the formation of this subcommittee was only recently announced during the course of our work. SAMHSA officials said that the new subcommittee under the BHCC will have an explicit focus on addressing serious mental illness, and that they expected this group to have an initial meeting in early 2015 to establish a direction for its forthcoming efforts. However, consistent with the BHCC, the subcommittee is only expected to coordinate within HHS, not across federal agencies.

Agency officials cited few specific actions taken by the coordination committees to address the needs of individuals with serious mental illness. For example, according to agency officials, the Psychological Health and Traumatic Brain Injury committee, co-chaired by DOD and VA, worked to implement the Integrated Mental Health Strategy, which the agencies jointly developed to address the mental health needs of servicemembers and veterans. However, VA officials said that none of the elements of this strategy or actions the committee has taken were specific to serious mental illness.

Table 3. Examples of Current Interagency Committees Related to Mental Health, Identified by Agency Officials

					Member agencies							
Committee name	**Year established**	**Meeting schedule**	**Target population**	**Goal**	**DOD**	**DOJ**	**DOL**	**Ed**	**HHS**	**HUD**	**SSA**	**VA**
Behavioral Health Coordinating Council	2010	Quarterly	Individuals with behavioral health issues	Share information and ensure that all behavioral health issues are being handled collaboratively and without duplication of effort across the agency					✓			
Interagency Task Force on Military and Veterans Mental Health[a]	2012	Quarterly	Veterans, service members, and their families with behavioral health issues	Coordinate and review agency efforts to enhance veteran and military mental health and substance abuse services and develop recommendations on strategies to improve mental health and substance abuse treatment services	✓			✓	✓			✓

Table 3. (Continued)

					Member agencies							
Committee name	**Year established**	**Meeting schedule**	**Target population**	**Goal**	**DOD**	**DOJ**	**DOL**	**Ed**	**HHS**	**HUD**	**SSA**	**VA**
United States Interagency Council on Homelessness[a]	1987	Quarterly	Individuals experiencing homelessness	Coordinate the federal response to homelessness and create a national partnership to reduce and end homelessness while maximizing the effectiveness of the federal government	✓	✓	✓	✓	✓	✓	✓	✓

Source: GAO analysis of agency information. | GAO-15-113

Legend:

DOD Department of Defense
DOJ Department of Justice
DOL Department of Labor
Ed Department of Education
HHS Department of Health and Human Services
HUD Department of Housing and Urban Development
SSA Social Security Administration
VA Department of Veterans Affairs

Note: Agency officials identified additional interagency committees that can support coordination but none were focused specifically on serious mental illness: the Coordinating Council on Juvenile Justice and Delinquency Prevention (DOD, DOJ, DOL, Education, HHS, HUD), the Curb Cuts to the Middle Class Initiative (DOJ, DOL, Education, HHS, SSA, VA), the DOD/VA Psychological Health and Traumatic Brain Injury Workgroup (DOD, VA), the Federal Interagency Reentry Council (DOJ, DOL, Education, HHS, HUD, SSA, VA), the Federal Working Group on Suicide Prevention (DOD, Education, HHS, VA), the Interagency Committee on Disability Research (Education, HHS, VA), the Now Is the Time Interagency Implementation Group (DOJ, Education, HHS), and the VA/Indian Health Service Post-Traumatic Stress Disorder Workgroup (HHS, VA). Some of these committees include additional agencies and/or organizations, not identified in this table.

[a]This committee includes additional agencies and/or organizations not identified in this table.

Although SAMHSA is charged with promoting coordination across the federal government regarding mental illness, its efforts to lead coordination—specifically on serious mental illness—across agencies have been lacking. According to SAMHSA's enabling legislation, as amended, it is required to promote coordination of programs relating to mental illness throughout the federal government.[39] In addition, SAMHSA's 2011-2014 strategic plan acknowledges the need for coordination, noting that no single program, either within HHS or anywhere else in the federal government, can solve the problems of homelessness, joblessness, educational challenges, and community cohesion for people with mental illness, including those with serious mental illness.[40] Despite SAMHSA's recognition of the need to coordinate, such coordination related to serious mental illness has been largely absent across the federal government. Further, our previous work has demonstrated the value of interagency coordination when it is supported by agency leadership. Without such coordination and support, agencies do not have the necessary information to assess the reach and effectiveness of their programs or to determine whether or where there may be gaps or overlap in services for individuals with serious mental illness.

Staff of Most Programs Specifically Targeting Individuals with Serious Mental Illness Reported Some Coordination

Although coordination specific to serious mental illness was lacking among interagency committees, staff who completed questionnaires regarding individual programs reported that they coordinate with their counterparts in other programs both within and across agencies.[41] Specifically, staff from 90 percent of the programs targeting serious mental illness (27 of 30 programs) reported coordinating with their counterparts in other programs.

Program staff reported via the questionnaire and in follow-up responses that they coordinated with other programs in the same agency. For example, according to SAMHSA officials, program staff from the mental health homelessness programs in SAMHSA's Center for Mental Health Services coordinated with staff in SAMHSA's Center for Substance Abuse Treatment in order to conduct a national evaluation of SAMHSA's homeless programs. This evaluation is a coordinated effort within SAMSHA to compare effectiveness of programs and models of service delivery such as those used by the Projects for Assistance in Transition from Homelessness program, which funded services in both community mental health and co-occurring alcohol and drug treatment. In another example, program staff from SAMHSA's Primary and Behavioral Health Care Integration program—a program that addresses the primary care needs of individuals with serious mental illness in an integrated community mental health center setting—reported collaborating with HHS's Health Resources and Services Administration to jointly fund a training and technical assistance center. According to staff for this program, the cooperative agreement targeted both the Primary and Behavioral Health Care Integration program grantees and the Health Resources and Services Administration's community health centers and has supported trainings, curricula development, and webinars.

In addition, program staff reported via the questionnaire and in follow-up responses that they have coordinated with programs in other agencies. Program staff from SAMHSA's Criminal and Juvenile Justice programs, for example, told us that they met quarterly with program staff for DOJ's Bureau of Justice Assistance Justice and Mental Health Collaboration program. They said that they strategized the use of resources at these meetings. While coordination at the program level is important to ensure that program staff are aware of the efforts of staff for other programs, it does not take the place of, or achieve the level of leadership, that we have noted in past work is key to successful coordination. Where programs to address an issue are spread across multiple agencies—as we have found they are in the case of serious mental illness—interagency coordination at the agency level can minimize the potential for duplication and overlap that could reduce the efficiency of federal programs. See appendix IV for more information on the coordination mechanisms and activities reported by program staff.

AGENCIES HAVE EVALUATED LESS THAN ONE-THIRD OF THE 30 PROGRAMS TARGETED FOR PEOPLE WITH SERIOUS MENTAL ILLNESS

Agencies completed few evaluations of the 30 programs that specifically targeted individuals with serious mental illness. Specifically, as of September 2014, 9 programs had a completed program evaluation, 4 programs had an evaluation underway, and 17 programs had no evaluation.[42] (See fig. 1.)

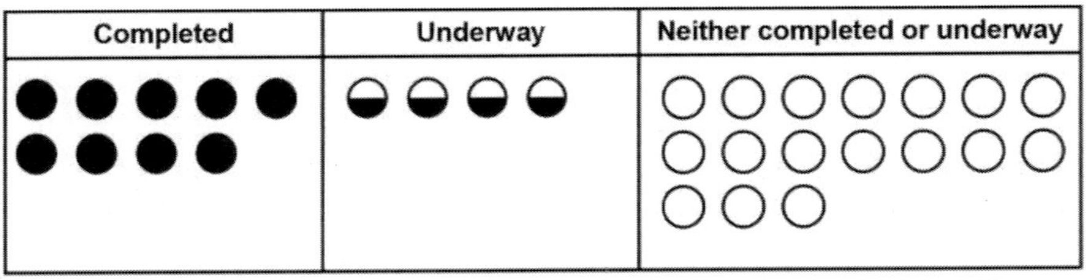

Source: GAO analysis of questionnaire responses from five federal agencies. | GAO-15-113.

Figure 1. Evaluation Status of 30 Federal Programs Targeting Individuals with Serious Mental Illness, as of September 2014.

Of the 9 completed program evaluations, 7 were completed by SAMHSA and 2 were completed by DOD. DOJ, SSA, and VA had not completed any evaluations for their targeted programs. Evaluations for both targeted DOD programs and two of the targeted SAMHSA programs were completed in 2013. Of the remaining 5, all of which are HHS's SAMHSA programs, 1 was completed in 2010, 2 were completed in 2011, and 2 were completed in 2014.

We found that these completed evaluations gave an overall assessment of the program, examined its strengths and weaknesses, and provided recommendations for improvement. For example, SAMHSA contracted with the Human Services Research Institute—a consulting and research firm—to conduct an evaluation of the Protection and Advocacy for Individuals with Mental Illness (PAIMI) program. Human Services Research Institute's 2011 evaluation report found that the program was successful in giving those with psychiatric disabilities a voice in the exercise of their rights, among other things. However, the report also found deficiencies in the program, such as insufficient training for federal program and contract officials regarding PAIMI requirements and frequent difficulties gaining access to at-risk individuals in residential settings. SAMHSA provided us with information about how the agency has addressed the deficiencies outlined in the PAIMI evaluation. In addition, the Army Deputy Chief of Staff conducted an evaluation of the Army National Guard Psychological Health program in 2013. The evaluation recommended that the program demonstrate that the services delivered were responding to a specific need of its target population—Army National Guard and Army Reservists—and noted that it is unclear whether the program is reaching Reservists. The evaluation also found that the program adhered to its quality standards and effectively solicited customer feedback. Four of the 30 programs targeting individuals with serious mental illness reported having evaluations underway that were scheduled for completion after September 2014. The SSA Homeless with Schizophrenia Presumptive Disability program is scheduled for completion in December 2014, the SAMHSA Projects for Assistance with the Transition from Homelessness program and Mental Health Homelessness Prevention programs are scheduled for completion in 2016, and the DOD Air Force Air National Guard Psychological Health program is scheduled for completion in 2017.

The remaining 17 programs targeting individuals with serious mental illness had not completed a program evaluation. This included all 3 DOJ programs, all 8 VA programs, 2 DOD programs, and 4 HHS programs. (See table 4.) Our prior work has shown that program evaluations address specific questions about program performance and may focus on assessing program operations or results. These evaluations can play a key role in agency strategic planning and in program management, providing important feedback on both program design and execution.[43] Although our past work has found that some program evaluations can be expensive, the relatively few evaluations completed among programs targeted for individuals with mental illness is a concern because without meaningful and timely evaluations, agencies may lose opportunities to identify improvements in federal government efficiency and effectiveness, and because comprehensive evaluations can be key to coordinating and streamlining federal programs.[44] See appendix V for a complete list of the 30 programs and their evaluation status.

Table 4. Evaluation Status of 30 Federal Programs Targeting Individuals with Serious Mental Illness, as of September 2014

Agency	Completed	Underway	None	Total
DOD	2	1	2	5
DOJ			3	3
HHS	7	2	4	13
SSA		1		1
VA			8	8
Total	9	4	17	30

Source: GAO analysis of questionnaire responses from five federal agencies. | GAO-15-113

Legend:

DOD Department of Defense

DOJ Department of Justice

HHS Department of Health and Human Services

SSA Social Security Administration

VA Department of Veterans Affairs

In some instances, agency officials provided explanations for the lack of completed program evaluations. For example, DOJ officials indicated that the Dual Diagnosis Residential Drug Abuse Program had not been evaluated because the number of participants was small; however, these officials told us that they would consider analyzing program effectiveness once a sufficient number of participants had been reached. SAMHSA officials noted that they considered a formal evaluation of the State and Community Partnerships to Integrate Services program but concluded that an evaluation could not be justified due to the high cost of such an evaluation relative to the size of the program. SAMHSA officials added, however, that the agency is conducting a consolidated evaluation of four of its homeless programs, including the Projects for Assistance with the Transition from Homelessness and Mental Health Homelessness Prevention programs. SAMHSA officials told us that in 2013, they established an evaluation team responsible for ensuring a centralized evaluation strategy and conducting evaluations of certain SAMHSA programs.

Agency officials also said they drew on evidence in the published literature to help ensure the effectiveness of their programs specifically targeting individuals with serious mental illness. Officials from several agencies told us they reviewed evidence-based articles in medical and scientific journals when considering treatment and services to provide to individuals with serious mental illness. For example, VA officials told us they consulted published literature and reviewed VA-generated data to help ensure program effectiveness in supporting those with serious mental illness. VA officials cited the agency's use of a specific drug for schizophrenic patients who have not responded to other antipsychotic medications; agency officials said they began using this treatment after reviewing published results of clinical trials using the drug in community settings. DOD officials said they followed a "hierarchy of reliable evidence" in determining interventions for individuals with mental health disorders and that clinical studies that contain scientifically valid data and are published in medical and scientific literature meet the requirements of reliable evidence. Finally, DOJ officials told us that they routinely reviewed the professional literature in peer-reviewed journals and consulted with experts to identify potential programs and services for individuals with serious mental illness.

In addition to relying on published research to help design programs that were effective, agency officials cited the use of ongoing monitoring and assessment activities for several of their programs targeting people with serious mental illness. For example, for the Specialized PTSD program, VA said they collected data from clinicians and program sites as veterans were admitted, treated, and discharged from services. The data were reviewed and aggregated and used to evaluate mandated reporting, workload, veteran characteristics and demographics, and the delivery of psychotherapy. In another example, HHS officials indicated they monitored program effectiveness by requiring recipients of grant and cooperative agreement programs to report program performance data. SAMHSA's strategic plan included specific performance and outcomes targets, including reductions in the percentage of individuals from ages 12 to 17 reporting major depression episodes in the past year and in the number of suicide attempts and deaths by suicide among high-risk populations.[45] While ongoing monitoring and reporting of program accomplishments, particularly progress toward established goals or standards, are essential to performance management, it cannot take the place of a formal program evaluation. We have reported previously on the importance of conducting program evaluations to inform program managers on the overall design and operation of the program.[46]

DOD officials also noted that in response to 2012 Executive Order 13625 on improving access to mental health services for veterans, servicemembers, and military families, they were reviewing all their mental health and substance use prevention, education, and outreach programs to identify the practices that produce the greatest impact on quality and outcomes and ranking the programs using metrics to assess their effectiveness. One document that DOD produced in January 2014 as a result of that review noted that, as a result of the Air Force Baseline Psychological Testing for Recruits program, trainees who stated during interviews that they were thinking of harming themselves or others were referred to a hospital emergency room for evaluation. The document suggested that these referrals may help reduce the number of suicides, but program officials also stated that the program's impact in this area cannot be measured because it is impossible to know if a trainee would have attempted suicide if they had not been referred.

CONCLUSION

Individuals with serious mental illness can face significant challenges getting the services they need. Agencies identified a wide range of federal programs—across multiple agencies—that can support individuals with serious mental illness. Although staff in programs targeting serious mental illness reported taking steps to coordinate their individual programs, coordination efforts among agency leadership to address serious mental illness are lacking. The absence of this high-level coordination hinders the federal government's ability to develop an overarching perspective of its programs supporting and targeting individuals with serious mental illness. Although SAMHSA—the agency within HHS that is required to promote coordination of programs relating to mental illness throughout the federal government—has made some effort to coordinate on mental health broadly, it has shown little leadership in coordinating federal efforts on behalf of those with serious mental illness. Without stronger leadership from HHS to coordinate an integrated, interagency approach, it is difficult to attain the type of high-level perspective needed to determine whether there are gaps in services. For example, federal agencies reported difficulty even identifying which programs can support this vulnerable population. Stronger HHS leadership can also help ensure that agencies have the necessary information to assess the reach and effectiveness of their programs for individuals with serious mental illness. The new subcommittee within HHS's BHCC may provide a useful starting point to facilitate this coordination around serious mental illness; however, the subcommittee is new and the BHCC is limited to HHS and is not an interagency committee.

We have also reported many times on the importance of conducting formal program evaluations to inform program managers on the overall design and operation of the program and ensure that the program's objectives are being met. Although about $5.7 billion was obligated by 4 agencies—DOD, HHS, DOJ, and VA—to support federal programs specifically targeting individuals with serious mental illnesses, less than one-third had a completed program evaluation. The public health, social, and economic impact of serious mental illness, coupled with the constrained fiscal environment of recent years, highlights the need to ensure that federal programs efficiently and effectively use their resources to support the complex needs of individuals with serious mental illness.

RECOMMENDATIONS

To understand the full breadth of federal programs and the scope of federal resources expended on programs supporting those with serious mental illness, we recommend that the Secretary of HHS establish a mechanism to facilitate intra- and interagency coordination, including actions that would assist with identifying the programs, resources, and potential gaps in federal efforts to support individuals with serious mental illness.

To help determine if programs are effective at supporting those individuals with serious mental illness, we recommend that the Secretaries of Defense, Health and Human Services, Veterans Affairs, and the Attorney General—which oversee programs targeting individuals with serious mental illness—document which of their programs targeted for individuals with serious mental illness should be evaluated and how often such evaluations should be completed.

AGENCY COMMENTS

We provided a draft of this report to DOD, DOJ, DOL, Education, HHS, HUD, SSA, and VA for review and comment. DOD, HHS, SSA, and VA provided written comments. DOJ, Education, HHS, and HUD provided technical comments on this report that we incorporated as appropriate. Although our report does not include recommendations directed to SSA, it said it agreed with our report. DOL had no comments on the report.

Our first recommendation was directed to HHS exclusively. HHS did not concur with this recommendation, which calls for the agency to establish a mechanism to facilitate intra- and interagency coordination. HHS noted that funding for SAMHSA is largely allocated to specific programs by Congress and thus improving coordination should include coordination at the Congressional level. HHS also stated that the recommendation was not supported because coordination was already occurring at the program level and there was not a specific need identified by agencies, stakeholders, or individuals with serious mental illness that more coordination was necessary.

The report acknowledges that coordination at a program level is important but notes that it cannot take the place of coordination at higher levels that would provide the perspective needed to assess the reach and effectiveness of all of the federal government's programs targeting individuals with serious mental illness. In addition, as we note in the report, SAMHSA's own enabling legislation, as amended, includes a requirement to promote coordination of programs relating to mental illness throughout the federal government, and its own strategic plan recognizes the need for coordination as well. In addition, our past work has highlighted the importance of interagency coordination supported by agency leadership. In light of these other sources demonstrating the importance of interagency coordination beyond the program staff level to the agency level, we believe our recommendation is appropriate and well-supported.

In addition, HHS expressed concern that we excluded Medicare and Medicaid from our scope, stating that this omission was unexplained and that it created inconsistencies in our findings because we included treatment and support services funded by DOD and VA. However, as we stated explicitly throughout the report, we excluded health benefit programs including Medicare, Medicaid, and TRICARE. The purpose of this report was to provide information on programs supporting individuals with serious mental illness beyond those of reimbursement. As a result, we do not believe it creates the inconsistencies stated by HHS. However, the draft included an estimate of spending on mental health services by Medicaid and Medicare to help address HHS's concern.

Our second recommendation on conducting program evaluations was directed to DOD, DOJ, HHS, and VA. HHS did not concur with this recommendation, while DOD, DOJ, and VA agreed. While HHS said that performance measurement is important, it stated that program evaluation is only one method of measurement and suggested that the report places undue importance on program evaluations in particular. In the report we acknowledge that there are other efforts to monitor performance and program effectiveness, including the performance and outcomes targets in SAMHSA's strategic plan, but as the report states, this type of ongoing monitoring cannot take the place of a program evaluation. In addition, HHS expressed concern that the report focused on completed evaluations, noting that some program evaluations provide interim results while still underway. In the report we acknowledge 2 HHS programs that have program evaluations underway. Therefore, we believe we have appropriately characterized the current status of the agency's program evaluations.

Linda T. Kohn
Director, Health Care

APPENDIX I: SCOPE AND METHODOLOGY

This appendix describes the methodology for developing, administering, and analyzing a web questionnaire for eight federal departments, agencies, and other entities to gather information on programs supporting individuals with serious mental illness or serious emotional disturbance, including any evaluation and coordination efforts undertaken related to those programs.[1]

Identification of Federal Agencies

To identify federal agencies that may have programs supporting individuals with serious mental illness or serious emotional disturbance, we reviewed the programs and agencies highlighted in the President's New Freedom Commission on Mental Health "Major Federal Programs Supporting and Financing Mental Health Care," reviewed our prior reports, other documents, such as reports from the Bazelon Center for Mental Health Law, and interviewed advocacy groups and agency officials.[2] Based on this review and our interviews, there were eight agencies that were cited frequently as having programs supporting individuals with serious mental illness, and we included those agencies in our review:

- Department of Defense (DOD)
- Department of Education (Education)
- Department of Health and Human Services (HHS)
- Department of Housing and Urban Development (HUD)
- Department of Justice (DOJ)
- Department of Labor (DOL)
- Department of Veterans Affairs (VA), and
- Social Security Administration (SSA).

Identification of Programs

To identify federal programs that support individuals with serious mental illness or serious emotional disturbance, we developed definitions to provide some clarity on the programs that should be included in our review. To develop these definitions, we examined applicable federal requirements, our prior work, and interviewed advocacy groups and federal officials. We defined the key terms as follows:

- **Program**: A federal program, activity, or initiative may include, but is not limited to, (1) grants to state, local, tribal, nonprofit, or research entities, (2) contracts with service providers, or (3) services directly provided to beneficiaries by the federal agency itself. This does not include health benefit programs—such as Medicaid, Medicare, or TRICARE—that reimburse providers for various mental health services.

- **Serious mental illness**: Adults who currently have, or at any time in the past year had, a diagnosable mental, behavioral, or emotional disorder (excluding developmental and substance use disorders) of sufficient duration to meet certain diagnostic criteria, as specified within the Diagnostic and Statistical Manual (DSM), that resulted in serious functional impairment, substantially interfering with or limiting one or more major life activities. Serious mental illness may also include individuals with a specific diagnosis, for example, individuals diagnosed with schizophrenia, schizoaffective disorder, bipolar disorder, or major depression.
- **Serious emotional disturbance**: Children and adolescents from birth up to age 18 who currently or at any time during the past year had, a diagnosable mental, behavioral, or emotional disorder of sufficient duration to meet diagnostic criteria specified within the DSM that resulted in functional impairment, which substantially interferes with or limits the child's role or functioning in family, school, or community activities. Serious emotional disturbance may also be a condition exhibiting one or more characteristics—such as a general pervasive mood of unhappiness or depression—over a long period of time and to a marked degree that adversely affects a child's educational performance as defined in the Individuals with Disabilities Education Act implementing regulations.[3]

We adopted these definitions to focus our review on programs that either directly administer or fund programs for the seriously mentally ill, as well as programs that may support a broader population likely to include those with serious mental illness. Given the wide range of programs included in this review, we relied on the federal agencies to identify the programs that met the criteria above. When necessary, we discussed these criteria with the agencies. For example, SAMHSA officials did not initially include any of their suicide prevention programs, submitting instead only those programs that were specifically targeted for individuals with serious mental illness. After several discussions, SAMHSA officials provided the names of 12 additional programs, including their suicide prevention programs that can provide general support to individuals with serious mental illness. However, SAMHSA officials did not identify the primary purpose or provide additional information on these more broadly focused programs.

We received requests from several agencies to eliminate some of their programs from our review for various reasons. For example, Navy and Marine Corps program staff included their substance abuse programs in their responses to the questionnaire. After discussions with DOD, we determined that since these programs focus on substance abuse rather than mental health they should be removed. We ultimately determined that it was appropriate to remove 13 programs from our review. In total, 112 programs were included in our final analysis.

Developing and Administering the Web-Based Questionnaire

We developed a web-based questionnaire to collect detailed information on federal programs that support individuals with serious mental illness or serious emotional disturbance for fiscal year 2013. It included questions on program goals, target groups served, evaluations conducted, and coordination activities with other federal agencies. In addition, the questionnaire asked agencies to identify which of these programs were specifically targeted for individuals with serious mental illness. We then verified this information through follow-ups with the agencies. Finally, the questionnaire also collected data on program obligations—defined as definite commitments that create a legal liability of the government for the payment of goods and services ordered or received—for fiscal year 2013. In some cases, we could not obtain data on funds obligated for these programs because agency officials told us that they did not report budgetary data at this level, among other reasons.

To minimize errors arising from differences in how questions may be interpreted, we conducted pretests with HHS and Education in February 2014. We made appropriate revisions and our final questionnaire was sent to several knowledgeable agency officials within each of the eight agencies. These officials were responsible for coordinating with the appropriate program staff to ensure we received completed questionnaires for these programs. Within the eight agencies, we received responses from program staff that were operating programs relevant to our purposes. The questionnaire was available from March 2014 to June 2014. In total, we received 44 completed questionnaires from program staff within the eight agencies. All eight agencies responded, for a 100 percent response rate.[4] We also made telephone calls to officials and sent them follow-up e-mail messages, as necessary, to clarify their responses or obtain additional information.

We used standard descriptive statistics to analyze responses to the questionnaire. Because this was not a sample survey, there were no sampling errors. To minimize other types of errors, commonly referred to as nonsampling errors, and to enhance data quality, we employed survey design practices in the development of the questionnaire and in the collection, processing, and analysis of the questionnaire data.

To reduce nonresponse, another source of nonsampling error, we sent out e-mail reminder messages and phone calls to encourage officials to complete the questionnaire. In reviewing the questionnaire data, we performed checks to identify inappropriate answers. We further reviewed the data for missing or ambiguous responses and followed up with agency officials when necessary to clarify their responses. As a result, we determined that the data used in this report were sufficiently reliable for our purposes.

Determining the Extent of Coordination

To assess coordination efforts among the higher levels of agency leadership, we reviewed information gathered through the questionnaire and interviewed agency officials from the agencies represented among the 30 programs—that is, those identified as targeting individuals with serious mental illness—regarding interagency committees established to facilitate coordination and collaboration. To determine the organizational structure, mission, and the actions taken by these committees, we also reviewed relevant interagency committee documents such as membership rosters, meeting agendas, and meeting minutes.

To assess coordination efforts at the program level, we used information gathered through the questionnaire to identify which of the 112 programs at the eight agencies included in our review had coordinated with other programs in an official capacity. Finally, we interviewed agency officials and reviewed relevant documentation related to the reported program-level coordination.

Assessing Evaluations

We used information gathered through the questionnaire to determine whether the eight agencies included in our review had begun or completed evaluations for any of their 112 programs. For the 30 programs that the agencies identified as targeting those with serious mental illness, we asked the agencies for copies of the most recent completed program evaluations. We reviewed the information provided to us to determine whether it met our definition of a program evaluation and, for each completed program evaluation, we reviewed its objectives and scope. Furthermore, we interviewed agency officials about factors affecting the lack of program evaluation. We also reviewed agency documents and interviewed agency officials to identify whether the agencies took other steps to help ensure that their programs are effective, such as whether the agencies used other methods—such as collecting outcome measures—to monitor their programs.

Appendix II: List of Programs That Can Support Individuals with Serious Mental Illness Identified by Eight Federal Agencies

Agency	Program name
Department of Defense[a]	InTransition
	National Intrepid Center of Excellence
	Non-medical counseling
	Patient-Centered Medical Home Behavioral Health
Air Force	Baseline Psychological Testing for Recruits
	Exceptional Family Member - Family Support
	Family Advocacy
	Suicide Prevention
	Tele-Behavioral Health
	Virtual Reality Exposure Therapy
	Wounded Warrior
Air National Guard	Psychological Health
Army	Behavioral Health System of Care
	Deployment Health Assessment
	Suicide Prevention
	Warrior Care and Transition
Army National Guard	Family Assistance Centers
	Psychological Health
	Suicide Prevention
Marine Corps[b]	Community Counseling
	Exceptional Family Member
	Family Advocacy
	Family Readiness
	Operational Stress Control and Readiness
	Suicide Prevention

Appendix II. (Continued)

Agency	Program name
	Wounded Warrior Regiment Call Center
	Wounded Warrior Regiment Medical Cell
Navy[b]	Back on Track
	Behavioral Health Needs Assessment Survey
	Families OverComing Under Stress
	Medical Case Management
	Overcoming Adversity and Stress Injury Support
	Special Psychiatric Response Intervention Team
	Suicide Prevention
Department of Education	
Office of Special Education and Rehabilitative Services	Centers for Independent Living[c]
	Individuals with Disabilities Education Act (IDEA) Part B
	IDEA Personnel Development
	IDEA Technical Assistance and Dissemination
	National Institute on Disability and Rehabilitation Research[c]
	State Independent Living Services[c]
	Vocational Rehabilitation Services
Department of Health and Human Services	
Administration for Community Living	Aging and Disability Resource Centers
	Alzheimer's Disease Supportive Services
	Home and Community-Based Supportive Services
Health Resources and Services Administration	Health Center Program
	National Health Service Corps
	Ryan White HIV/AIDS Program
Indian Health Service	Mental Health/Social Services
National Institutes of Health	Scientific Research
Substance Abuse and Mental Health Services Administration[d]	American Indian/Alaska Native Suicide Prevention Initiative
	Children and Family Programs
	Community Mental Health Services Block Grant
	Consumer and Consumer Support Technical Assistance
	Criminal and Juvenile Justice Programs
	Disaster Response
	Garrett Lee Smith Youth Suicide Prevention – States
	Garrett Lee Smith Youth Suicide Prevention – Campus
	HIV/AIDS Education
	Mental Health Homelessness Prevention
	Mental Health Transformation Grant
	Minority HIV/AIDS
	Practice Improvement and Training
	Primary and Behavioral Health Care Integration

Agency	Program name
	Project LAUNCH
	Projects for Assistance in Transition from Homelessness
	Protection and Advocacy for Individuals with Mental Illness
	Seclusion and Restraint and Trauma
	State and Community Partnerships to Integrate Services
	Statewide Consumer Network
	Statewide Family Network
	Suicide Lifeline
	Suicide Prevention Resource
	System of Care Expansion Implementation Cooperative
	Youth Violence Prevention
Department of Housing and Urban Development	
Office of Community Planning and Development	Continuum of Care
	Emergency Solutions Grant
	Housing Opportunities for Person with AIDS
Office of Housing	Section 811 Supportive Housing for Person with Disabilities
Office of Public and Indian Housing	HUD-VA Supportive Housing
Department of Justice	
Bureau of Justice Assistance	Justice and Mental Health Collaboration
	Second Chance Act Reentry
Bureau of Prisons	Mental Health Step Down Unit
	Dual Diagnosis Residential Drug Abuse
	Resolve
	Steps Toward Awareness, Growth, and Emotional Strength
	Skills Program
Office of Juvenile Justice and Delinquency Prevention	Family Juvenile Drug Court
	Formula Grant
	Juvenile Accountability Block Grant
	Second Chance Act Reentry
Department of Labor	
Employment and Training Administration	Disability Employment Initiative
	Reintegration of Ex-Offenders
	Workforce Investment Act Youth Activities
	YouthBuild
Office of Disability Employment Policy	Disability.gov
	Job Accommodation Network
	Workforce Recruitment Program
Veterans' Employment and Training Service	Homeless Veterans Reintegration Program
Social Security Administration	

Appendix II. (Continued)

Agency	Program name
Office of Retirement and Disability Policy	Homeless with Schizophrenia Presumptive Disability
	Military Casualties/Wounded Warriors
	Protection and Advocacy
	Work Incentives Planning and Assistance
Department of Veterans Affairs	
Veterans Health Administration	General Outpatient Mental Health Services
	Inpatient Mental Health
	Intensive Community Mental Health Recovery
	Mental Health Residential Rehabilitation Treatment
	Primary Care Mental Health Integration
	Psychosocial Rehabilitation and Recovery Center
	Re-Engaging Veterans with Serious Mental Illness
	Specialized Homeless Services[e]
	Specialized Post-Traumatic Stress Disorder
	Substance Use Disorder Treatment
	Therapeutic and Supported Employment Services

Source: GAO analysis of questionnaire responses and interviews with eight federal agencies. | GAO-15-113

Notes: The scope of this report did not include health benefit programs—such as Medicaid, Medicare, and TRICARE—that reimburse providers for various mental health services.

[a] DOD officials said they experienced difficulty in identifying all the programs that may generally support individuals with serious mental illness and acknowledged that there could be other programs that support this population but are not included in this list.

[b] In addition to the programs listed in this table, the Marine Corps and the Navy each initially included in their questionnaire responses their substance abuse and rehabilitation programs, which officials described as providing treatment for, among other things, co-occurring conditions, which may include serious mental illness. However, DOD officials informed us that the Army had a similar program that was not included in their questionnaire responses, and asked us to remove the Marine Corps and Navy programs to ensure consistency in the programs identified across the services.

[c] The Workforce Innovation and Opportunity Act, enacted on July 22, 2014, provides for the transfer of the functions related to the Centers for Independent Living program, State Independent Living program, and National Institute on Disability, Independent Living, and Rehabilitation Research from the Department of Education to the Administration for Community Living at the Department of Health and Human Services, envisioning an orderly transition period to effectuate the transferred authorities. Pub. L. No. 113-128, tit. IV, §§ 491, 503(e), 506(d), 128 Stat. 1425, 1695, 1701-1705 (July 22, 2014).

[d] In addition to completing the questionnaire for 13 programs SAMHSA administers that are targeted to individuals with serious mental illness, SAMHSA officials also provided the names of 12 programs that can offer general support to individuals with serious mental illness.

[e] This program includes the jointly administered Department of Housing and Urban Development's and Department of Veterans Affair's Supportive Housing Program, among others.

APPENDIX III: LIST OF PROGRAMS SPECIFICALLY TARGETING INDIVIDUALS WITH SERIOUS MENTAL ILLNESS IDENTIFIED BY EIGHT FEDERAL AGENCIES

Agency	Program name	Program description	Population served	Fiscal year 2013obligations
Department of Defense				
Air Force	Baseline Psychological Testing for Recruits	A screening program completed during basic military training at Joint Base San Antonio to identify mental health and behavioral problems.	Servicemembers	$800,000a
	Virtual Reality Exposure Therapy	Selected Air Force medical treatment facilities are outfitted with interactive virtual reality systems for use in enhanced exposure therapy between behavioral health providers and patients suffering from conditions such as post-traumatic stress disorder (PTSD), mild traumatic brain injury, addictions, phobias, and anger management issues.	Servicemembers	280,000
Air National Guard	Psychological Health Program	Provides assessment services, ensures continuity and engagement in treatment, and prevents servicemembers from falling through the cracks. This program does not provide direct treatment services.	Servicemembers and their families	14,460,000

Appendix III. (Continued)

Agency	Program name	Program description	Population served	Fiscal year 2013obligations
Army National Guard	Psychological Health Program	Provides assessment services, ensures continuity and engagement in treatment, and prevents servicemembers from falling through the cracks. This program does not provide direct treatment services.	Servicemembers and their families	14,400,000
Navy	Overcoming Adversity and Stress Injury Support	This is a 10-week comprehensive residential treatment program for Active Duty members with combat related stress disorders, including PTSD. Includes evidence-based treatment such as cognitive processing therapy, along with psychopharmacological interventions and complementary alternative treatments.	Servicemembers	1,132,630
Department of Health and Human Services				
Substance Abuse and Mental Health Services Administration	Community Mental Health Services Block Grant	Distributes funding to eligible states and territories for a variety of mental health prevention and treatment services; planning; administration; and educational activities under the state plan for comprehensive community-based mental health services for children with serious emotional disturbance and adults with serious mental illness.	Children and youth (birth to age 17), adults (age 18-64)	463,808,709b

Agency	Program name	Program description	Population served	Fiscal year 2013obligations
	Consumer and Consumer Support Technical Assistance	Provides support for technical assistance to facilitate the restructuring of the mental health system by promoting consumer directed approaches for adults with serious mental illness.	Adults	1,775,174b
	Criminal and Juvenile Justice	Diverts individuals with serious mental illness from the criminal justice system by providing support services that connect the individual to behavioral health, housing, and job placement services.	Incarcerated or previously incarcerated individuals, veterans	4,753,521b
	Mental Health Homelessness Prevention	Provides comprehensive services focusing on outreach, engagement, intensive case management, mental health services, substance abuse treatment, benefits support, and linkage to permanent housing.	Chronically homeless individuals, families	23,017,648b
	Mental Health Transformation Grant	Supports state and local governments creation or capacity expansion of evidence-based practices addressing the prevention of mental illness; trauma-informed care; screening, treatment and support services for military personnel; and housing and employment support.	Homeless individuals, Incarcerated or previously incarcerated, persons with HIV/AIDS, veterans	8,550,921b

Appendix III. (Continued)

Agency	Program name	Program description	Population served	Fiscal year 2013obligations
	Minority HIV/AIDS	Expands behavioral health services to individuals who are at risk for or have serious mental illness and/or co-occurring substance use disorder and are at risk or living with HIV/AIDS. Supports programs that develop or expand behavioral health and primary care networks in order to reduce the impact of behavioral health problems, HIV risk and HIV-related health disparities.	Individuals with HIV/AIDS	7,340,027b
	Primary and Behavioral Health Care Integration	Funds the coordination and integration of primary care services into publicly-funded community behavioral health settings. The program encourages grantees to engage in necessary partnerships, expand infrastructure and increase the availability of primary health care and wellness services to individuals with mental illness.	Adults, clderly (age 65 or older)	28,857,978b

Agency	Program name	Program description	Population served	Fiscal year 2013obligations
	Projects for Assistance in Transition from Homelessness	Supports services and resources to people with serious mental illness, including those with co-occurring substance use disorder, who are experiencing homelessness or at risk for homelessness. Provides funds for community-based outreach, case management, screening and diagnostic treatment, alcohol or drug treatment, and a limited set of housing services.	Homeless individuals, Individuals at-risk of homelessness	61,405,176b
	Protection and Advocacy for Individuals with Mental Illness	Provides grant awards to support protection and advocacy systems designated by the governor of each state or mayor of the District of Columbia. These systems monitor compliance with the Constitution and federal and state laws within public and private residential care, treatment facilities, and non-medical community-based facilities for individuals with serious mental illness, children, and youth.	Children and youth, adults	33,571,479b

Appendix III. (Continued)

Agency	Program name	Program description	Population served	Fiscal year 2013obligations
	State and Community Partnerships to Integrate Services	Supports the creation of developmentally appropriate local systems of care to improve outcomes of youth and young adults with serious mental health conditions. The grants fund integration of local systems with state, tribal, or territorial levels in areas such as education, employment, housing, mental health and co-occurring disorders, and decrease contacts with the juvenile and criminal system.	Young adults (ages 16-25)	2,929,027b
	Statewide Consumer Network	Provides funding to consumer-driven organizations to enhance statewide service system capacity. Promotes skill development, business management, and partnership building as part of the recovery process for mental health consumers.	Adults	2,093,606b
	Statewide Family Network	Provides information, referrals, and support at the state and local level to families who have a child with a serious emotional disturbance.	Children and youth, families	2,810,000b

Agency	Program name	Program description	Population served	Fiscal year 2013obligations
	System of Care Expansion Implementation Cooperative	Supports broad-scale operation, expansion and integration of systems of care to improve behavioral outcomes of children and youth with serious emotional disturbances and their families.	Children and youth, families	92,084,766b
Department of Justice				164,200,000c
Bureau of Prisons	Dual Diagnosis Residential Drug Abuse Program	An intensive residential substance abuse treatment program providing services for inmates with co-occurring substance use disorders and serious mental illnesses. The program is 9-months, unit-based, and offers cognitive-behavioral interventions in a modified therapeutic community setting.	Incarcerated adults	c
	Mental Health Step Down Unit	Offers an intermediate level of care for inmates with serious mental illness who do not require inpatient treatment, but lack the skills to function independently in a general population prison. Programs operate as modified therapeutic communities and utilize cognitive behavioral treatments, cognitive rehabilitation, and skills training.	Incarcerated adults	c

Appendix III. (Continued)

Agency	Program name	Program description	Population served	Fiscal year 2013obligations
	Steps Toward Awareness, Growth, and Emotional Strength	A unit-based residential psychology treatment program that focuses on inmates with serious mental illness and a primary diagnosis of Borderline Personality Disorder. Uses evidence-based treatments to increase time between disruptive behaviors and increase pro-social skills, and aims to prepare inmates for transition to less secure prison settings or promote successful reentry to socicty.	Incarcerated adults	c
Social Security Administration				
Office of Retirement and Disability Policy	Homeless with Schizophrenia Presumptive Disability	Aims to remove barriers to supplemental security income for individuals who have been diagnosed with schizophrenia or schizoaffective disorder who are known to be homeless by helping them through the application process and providing presumptive disability payments.	Homeless adults	N/Ad

Agency	Program name	Program description	Population served	Fiscal year 2013obligations
Department of Veterans Affairs (VA)				
Veterans Health Administration	Intensive Community Mental Health Recovery	Provides veterans with serious mental illness intensive recovery-oriented mental health services in their home and community that enable them to live in the community of their choosing. Connects veterans with a team that may include peer specialists, social workers, psychologists and physicians.	Veterans	142,532,724
	Mental Health Residential Rehabilitation Treatment	Provides residential rehabilitation and treatment services for veterans with mental health and substance use disorders, medical conditions and psychosocial needs, such as homelessness and unemployment. The program addresses the goals of rehabilitation, recovery, and community integration. It provides specific treatment for mental health, substance use disorders and medical conditions.	Veterans	858,119,000
	Psychosocial Rehabilitation and Recovery Center	Supports recovery and integration into the community for veterans with serious mental illness and severe functional impairment. Includes individual assessment and curriculum planning, skills training classes, family education programs, psychiatric services, compensated work therapy, and case management services.	Veterans	77,307,206

Appendix III. (Continued)

Agency	Program name	Program description	Population served	Fiscal year 2013obligations
	Re-Engaging Veterans with Serious Mental Illness	Identifies veterans with schizophrenia or bipolar disorder who have received care but have been lost to follow-up (no outpatient visits and no inpatient visits of more than 2 days) for at least 1 year. Contact information of identified veterans are sent to a social worker or psychologist at VA medical centers and community outpatient clinics who make efforts to locate, contact, assess the needs, and invite the veterans to return to care.	Veterans	e
	Specialized PTSD	Provides a range of inpatient and outpatient treatments for veterans diagnosed with military-based PTSD. These services use psychotherapies and psychopharmacology. Examples of specialty PTSD inpatient treatment are: Domiciliary PTSD, Women's Trauma Recovery Program. Specialty PTSD outpatient treatment includes Substance Use PTSD and Women's Stress Disorder Treatment Team.	Veterans	372,364,000

Agency	Program name	Program description	Population served	Fiscal year 2013obligations
	Therapeutic and Supported Employment Services	A continuum of recovery-oriented vocational rehabilitation programs that help veterans with mental health disabilities (including individuals with co-occurring physical disabilities) and a history of occupational dysfunction overcome barriers to employment and return to the workforce.	Veterans	133,747,000
	VA Specialized Homeless Services	A continuum of care designed to assist eligible homeless veterans and veterans at risk for homelessness. Services include homelessness prevention and rapid re-housing; assistance to veterans involved with the justice system; community case management; and employment assistance.	Homeless adults, veterans	1,404,890,000
	Inpatient Mental Health	Provides services to veterans with acute and severe emotional and/or behavioral symptoms that may cause a safety risk to the self or others, and/or may result in severely compromised functional status, including veterans with serious mental illness. Programs provide a range of intensive clinical services (e.g., close safety monitoring, close medication management) and frequent group therapy and psychoeducation.	Veterans	1,766,716,000

Source: GAO analysis of questionnaire responses. | GAO-15-113

Legend:

HUD Department of Housing and Urban Development

PTSD post-traumatic stress disorder

VA Department of Veterans Affairs

Notes:

[a]This amount only includes the analytic component. The amount for the clinical component is unknown.

[b]This amount only includes the obligated funds for the grants, not the obligated amount for the overall program.

[c]This amount includes all services and programs offered through Department of Justice's Psychology Services departments. These departments provide routine mental health screening, evaluation, brief counseling, individual therapy, group therapy, and crisis intervention. Psychology Services departments also provide specialty programming for specific populations.

[d]This was a pilot program designed and operated internally by Social Security Administration staff, with assistance from partner agencies in the involved communities. There was no obligated funding for this program in fiscal year 2013.

[e]Case identification was through the Serious Mental Illness Treatment Resource and Evaluation Center. Subsequently, targeted outreach was conducted at local medical centers and clinics as part of the overall program of care for veterans with serious mental illness.

APPENDIX IV: QUESTIONNAIRE RESPONSES ON COORDINATION FOR PROGRAMS TARGETING INDIVIDUALS WITH SERIOUS MENTAL ILLNESS

Program staff in the 30 programs targeting individuals with serious mental illness reported using a variety of coordination mechanisms and activities when working with other programs both within and across agencies.1As reported by program staff, the most frequent program-level coordinating mechanisms used were participating in an intra- or interagency committee or taskforce (11 programs) or developing or sharing tools that facilitate collaboration—for example, shared databases (10 programs). (See fig. 2.)

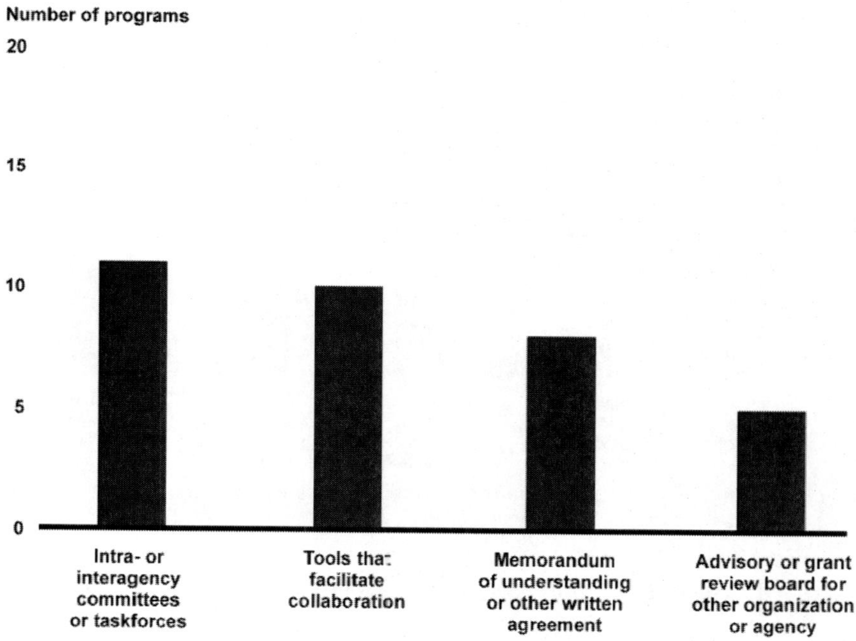

Source: GAO analysis of questionnaire responses from five federal agencies. | GAO-15-113.

Note: Tools that facilitate collaboration include, for example, shared databases and web portals.

Figure 2. Mechanisms Used When Coordinating in an Official Capacity in Fiscal Year 2013, as Reported by Program Staff.

Referral of patients or clients was the most frequently cited coordination activity for programs targeting individuals with serious mental illness (see fig. 3). For example, program staff for the Department of Justice's Bureau of Prisons' Dual Diagnosis Residential Drug Abuse Program received referrals after inmates have been pre-screened by Bureau of Priso

Designations and Sentence Computations Center. Involving other agencies in strategic planning was the second most commonly reported coordination activity by program staff (12 programs).

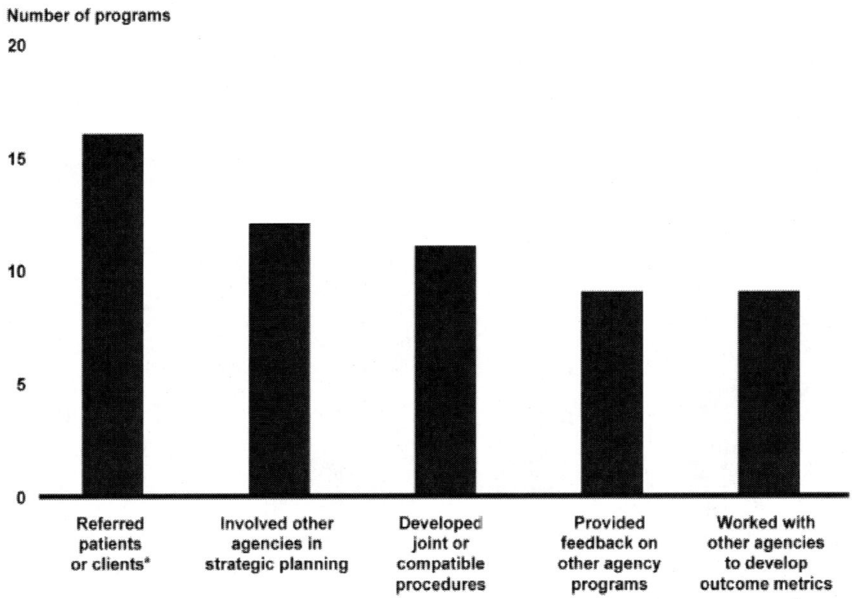

Source: GAO analysis of questionnaire responses from five federal agencies. | GAO-15-113.

[a] Substance Abuse and Mental Health Services Administration officials noted that they do not directly make referrals but fund grantees that may provide these services.

Figure 3. Coordination Activities Program Staff Participated in an Official Capacity in Fiscal Year 2013, as Reported by Program Staff.

Appendix V: Status of Evaluations of Federal Programs Targeting Individuals with Serious Mental Illness, as of September 2014

Agency	Program name	Completed or underway evaluation (Y/N)	Year completed or scheduled completion
Department of Defense			
Air Force	Baseline Psychological Testing for Recruits	Y	2013
	Virtual Reality Exposure Therapy	N	
Air National Guard	Psychological Health Program	Y	2017
Army National Guard	Psychological Health Program	Y	2013
Navy	Overcoming Adversity and Stress Injury Support	Na	
Department of Health and Human Services			
Substance Abuse and Mental Health Service Administration	Community Mental Health Services Block Grant	Y	2010
	Consumer and Consumer Support Technical Assistance	N	
	Criminal and Juvenile Justice	Y	2014
	Mental Health Homelessness Prevention	Y	2016
	Mental Health Transformation Grant	Y	2011
	Minority HIV/AIDS	Y	2014
	Primary and Behavioral Health Care Integration	Y	2013
	Projects for Assistance in Transition from Homeless	Y	2016
	Protection and Advocacy for Individuals with Mental Illness	Y	2011
	State and Community Partnerships to Integrate Services	N	

Appendix V. (Continued)

Agency	Program name	Completed or underway evaluation (Y/N)	Year completed or scheduled completion
	Statewide Consumer Network	N	
	Statewide Family Network	N	
	System of Care Expansion Implementation Cooperative	Y	2013
Department of Justice			
Bureau of Prisons	Mental Health Step Down Unit	N	
	Dual Diagnosis Residential Drug Abuse	N	
	Steps Toward Awareness, Growth, and Emotional Strength	N	
Social Security Administration			
Office of Retirement and Disability Policy	Homeless with Schizophrenia Presumptive Disability	Y	2014
Department of Veterans Affairs			
Veterans Health Administration	Intensive Community Mental Health Recovery	N	
	Mental Health Residential Rehabilitation Treatment	N	
	Psychosocial Rehabilitation and Recovery Center	N	
	Re-Engaging Veterans with Serious Mental Illness	N	
	Specialized PTSD	N	
	Therapeutic and Supported Employment Services	N	

Agency	Program name	Completed or underway evaluation (Y/N)	Year completed or scheduled completion
	Specialized Homeless Services	N	
	Inpatient Mental Health	N	

Source: GAO analysis of questionnaire responses from five federal agencies. | GAO-15-113

Note:

[a] Navy staff noted that they conducted an internal review of this program completed in June 2014; however, they did not provide any documentation related to this review.

End Notes

[1] Data are from the 2013 National Survey on Drug Use and Health, a national survey administered by SAMHSA.

[2] For the purposes of this report, we define individuals with serious mental illness as adults who currently or at any time in the past year have had a diagnosable mental, behavioral, or emotional disorder (excluding developmental and substance use disorders) of sufficient duration to meet certain diagnostic criteria, as specified within the Diagnostic and Statistical Manual of Mental Disorders (DSM), that resulted in serious functional impairment, substantially interfering with or limiting one or more major life activities. Individuals with serious mental illness may also include those with a specific diagnosis; for example, individuals diagnosed with schizophrenia, schizoaffective disorder, bipolar disorder, or major depression. In addition, we defined individuals with serious emotional disturbance as children and adolescents from birth up to age 18 who currently or at any time during the past year have had a diagnosable mental, behavioral, or emotional disorder of sufficient duration to meet diagnostic criteria specified within DSM that resulted in functional impairment, which substantially interferes with or limits the child's role or functioning in family, school, or community activities. Throughout this report, when we refer to programs generally supporting or specifically targeting individuals with serious mental illness, we are referring to programs supporting or targeting individuals with either serious mental illness or serious emotional disturbance.

[3] Data are from the 2013 National Survey on Drug Use and Health, a national survey administered by SAMHSA.

[4] OMB, *Letter from OMB Director Burwell to Chairman Murphy and Ranking Member DeGette, Subcommittee on Oversight and Investigations, House Energy and Commerce Committee,* November 7, 2013. Accessed October 21, 2014, http://energycommerce.house.gov/sites/republicans.energycommerce.house.gov/files/lette rs/MentalHealth/20131107OMB-MH-Inventory-Response.pdf.

[5] GAO, *Managing for Results: Implementation Approaches Used to Enhance Collaboration in Interagency Groups,* GAO-14-220 (Washington, D.C.: Feb. 14, 2014).

[6] We defined a federal program as a program, activity, or initiative that may include, but is not limited to, (1) grants to state, local, tribal, nonprofit, or research entities, (2) contracts with service providers, or (3) services directly provided to beneficiaries by the federal agency itself. We excluded health benefit programs—such as Medicaid, Medicare, or TRICARE—that may reimburse for various mental health services.

[7] For the purposes of this report, we refer to those federal departments, agencies, and other federal entities included in our scope as "agencies."

[8] The eight federal agencies selected for the web-based questionnaire were Department of Defense, Department of Education, HHS, Department of Housing and Urban Development, Department of Justice, Department of Labor, Social Security Administration, and Department of Veterans Affairs.

[9] Mental disorders are diagnosed using criteria in the Diagnostic and Statistical Manual of Mental Disorders—Fifth Edition (DSM-V). Each diagnosis, such as generalized anxiety disorder, major depressive disorder, or schizophrenia, is based on a specific set of symptoms reported over a given period of time. For example, major depressive disorder can be diagnosed if an individual reports experiencing five or more of nine specified symptoms, such as fatigue, feelings of worthlessness or excessive or inappropriate guilt, and a diminished ability to concentrate, over a minimum of 2 weeks.

[10] Substance Abuse and Mental Health Services Administration, *Leading Change: A Plan for SAMHSA's Roles and Actions 2011-2014*, HHS Publication No. (SMA) 11-4629 (Rockville, Md.: 2011).

[11] We are currently examining SAMHSA's Center for Mental Health Service's oversight of selected mental health grant programs.

[12] We define coordination as any joint effort that is intended to produce more public value than could be produced when organizations act alone. Fragmentation refers to those circumstances in which more than one federal agency is involved in the same broad area of national need and opportunities exist to improve service delivery.

[13] GAO, *Managing for Results: Key Considerations for Implementing Interagency Collaborative Mechanisms*, GAO-12-1022 (Washington, D.C.: Sept. 27, 2012).

[14] GAO, *Government Efficiency and Effectiveness: Opportunities to Reduce Fragmentation, Overlap, and Duplication through Enhanced Performance Management and Oversight*, GAO-13-590T (Washington, D.C.: May 22, 2013).

[15] GAO, *Designing Evaluations: 2012 Revision*, GAO-12-208G (Washington, D.C.: January 2012).

[16] Pub. L. No. 103-62, 107 Stat. 285 (Aug. 3, 1993), as expanded by Pub. L. No. 111-352, 124 Stat. 3866 (Jan. 4, 2011).

[17] One of HUD's programs, HUD-VA Supportive Housing, is co-administered by VA, which also submitted the program through the questionnaire. To avoid double-counting, this program is included only once in the overall total, but is listed twice in app. II, which details the programs.

[18] The questionnaire asked agencies to identify those programs that may support individuals with serious mental illness, with a question asking them to identify—within the supportive programs—those specific programs that are targeted for individuals with serious mental illness. For the purposes of the questionnaire, we defined a federal program as any program, activity, or initiative that may include, but is not limited to, (1) grants to state, local, tribal, nonprofit, or research entities, (2) contracts with service providers, or (3) services directly provided to beneficiaries by the federal agency itself.

[19] SAMHSA officials completed the questionnaire for 13 programs they administer. Subsequently, SAMHSA officials provided the names of an additional 12 programs that can offer general support to individuals with serious mental illness.

[20] Agency officials told us that, in general, they did not target their programs to individuals with specific serious mental illnesses, such as schizophrenia or bipolar disorder.

[21] Although agencies reported a single primary purpose for their programs, it is possible that some programs provide more than one service. For example, according to HHS officials the Community Mental Health Services Block Grant program provides funding to states for support and treatment services.

[22] This number only includes the reported obligated amounts for the 30 targeted programs and does not include other programs that individuals with serious mental illness may access, such as some homeless service programs, which are not specifically targeted for individuals with serious mental illness.

[23] This amount does not include health benefit programs—such as TRICARE—that may reimburse providers for various mental health services.

[24] SAMSHA officials only provided the obligated amount for the grants, not the full obligated amount for the program.

[25] The scope of this report did not include programs that may reimburse providers for mental health services, such as Medicaid and Medicare. OMB reported that, for fiscal year 2012, the federal spending on mental health services through Medicaid—a joint federal and state health care program—and Medicare was approximately $40 billion.

[26] DOJ could not provide the obligated funding specific to the three targeted programs. The obligated amount in this estimate included all services and programs offered through DOJ's Psychology Services departments. DOJ's Psychology Services departments provide routine mental health screening, evaluation, grief counseling, individual therapy, group therapy, and crisis intervention. DOJ's Psychology Services departments also provide specialty programming for specific populations.

[27] The Workforce Innovation and Opportunity Act, enacted on July 22, 2014, provides for the transfer of the functions related to the Centers for Independent Living program, State Independent Living program, and National Institute on Disability, Independent Living, and Rehabilitation Research from the Department of Education to the Administration for Community Living at the Department of Health and Human Services, envisioning an orderly transition period to effectuate the transferred authorities. Pub. L. No. 113-128, tit. IV, §§ 491, 503(e), 506(d), 128 Stat. 1425, 1695, 1701-1705 (July 22, 2014).

[28] Pub. L. No. 111-352, § 7, 124 Stat. 3866, 3876 (Jan. 4, 2011).

[29] GAO, *Government Efficiency and Effectiveness: Views on the Progress and Plans for Addressing Government-wide Management Challenges*, GAO-14-436T (Washington, D.C.: Mar. 12, 2014).

[30] National Institutes of Health officials told us that grants included in the Scientific Research program are publically reported on their website, see http://report.nih.gov.

[31] For the purposes of the questionnaire, we defined a federal program as a program, activity, or initiative that may include, but is not limited to, (1) grants to state, local, tribal, nonprofit, or research entities, (2) contracts with service providers, or (3) services directly provided to beneficiaries by the federal agency itself.

[32] National Institutes of Health is made up of 27 institutes and centers, one of which is the National Institute of Mental Health. Officials indicated that mental health research activities may be supported by various institutes and centers.

[33] We asked agencies to identify programs targeted specifically for individuals with serious mental illness as well as programs that may support that population, though not exclusively. For example, we asked agencies to include programs such as those that target the homeless population, as many of those individuals may suffer from serious mental illness.

[34] GAO-14-436T.

[35] Our previous work has identified the establishment of interagency groups as a mechanism for implementing coordination efforts. See GAO, *Managing for Results: Key Considerations for Implementing Interagency Collaborative Mechanisms*, GAO-12-1022 (Washington, D.C.: Sept. 27, 2012). In this report we refer to these groups as committees.

[36] GAO, *Young Adults With Serious Mental Illness: Some States and Federal Agencies Are Taking Steps to Address Their Transition Challenges,* GAO-08-678 (Washington, D.C.: June 23, 2008).

[37] The BHCC had six subcommittees that addressed selected topics, and three of these subcommittees specifically address substance use. One of the six subcommittees has done work that was related to serious mental illness, based on information HHS provided on recent actions taken by the BHCC.

[38] The Interagency Task Force was established by executive order. Improving Access to Mental Health Services for Veterans, Servicemembers, and Military Families, Executive Order No. 13625, 77 Fed. Reg. 54783 (Aug. 31, 2012).

[39] 42 U.S.C. § 290aa(d)(18).

[40] Substance Abuse and Mental Health Services Administration, *Leading Change*. SAMHSA has also released their strategic plan for 2015-2018: Substance Abuse and Mental Health Services Administration, *Leading Change 2.0: Advancing the Behavioral Health of the Nation 2015-2018,* HHS Publication No. (PEP) 14-LEADCHANGE2, 2014 (Rockville, Md.: 2014).

[41] In addition to the responses received via the questionnaire, we obtained further details via follow-up questions.

[42] We define program evaluation to be an individual, systematic study to assess how well a program or programs are working.

[43] GAO-12-208G.

[44] For example, we previously reported on a government-wide survey that we conducted in 2013. It showed that only 37 percent of all federal managers reported that, for the programs with which they had been involved, an evaluation had been completed within the last 5 years. We also found that 80 percent of managers surveyed whose programs did have evaluations reported that they contributed to a moderate or greater extent to improving program management or performance and to assessing program effectiveness or value. See GAO, *Program Evaluation: Strategies to Facilitate Agencies' Use of Evaluation in Program Management and Policy Making*, GAO-13-570 (Washington, D.C.: June 26, 2013); *Managing for Results: 2013 Federal Managers Survey on Organizational Performance and Management Issues*, GAO-13-519SP (Washington, D.C.: June 26, 2013); and GAO-12-208G.

[45] Substance Abuse and Mental Health Services Administration, *Leading Change*, and *Leading Change 2.0*. The new strategic plan also includes these targets.

[46] GAO-12-208G.

End Notes for Appendix I

[1] For the purposes of the report, we refer to those federal departments, agencies, and other entities included in our scope as "agencies." In addition, when we refer to programs generally supporting or specifically targeting individuals with serious mental illness, we are referring to programs supporting or targeting individuals with either serious mental illness or serious emotional disturbance.

[2] The President's New Freedom Commission on Mental Health, *Major Federal Programs Supporting and Financing Mental Health Care.* (Rockville, Md.: January 2003).

[3] See 34 C.F.R. § 300.8(a)(4).

[4] After some discussion with the National Institutes of Health, it was determined that it would provide information on its mental health project grants through interviews and other documentation rather than the web-based questionnaire.

End Note for Appendix IV

[1] Our past work has identified a range of mechanisms or strategies that the federal government uses to lead and implement interagency coordination, including interagency groups.

In: Federal Programs
Editor: Benjamin Wright

ISBN: 978-1-63483-043-0

Chapter 2

TESTIMONY OF RICHARD G. FRANK, ASSISTANT SECRETARY FOR PLANNING AND EVALUATION, U.S. DEPARTMENT OF HEALTH AND HUMAN SERVICES. HEARING ON "FEDERAL EFFORTS ON MENTAL HEALTH: WHY GREATER HHS LEADERSHIP IS NEEDED"*

Chairman Murphy, Ranking Member DeGette and members of the Subcommittee, thank you for this opportunity to discuss how the Department of Health and Human Services (HHS) is supporting the needs of people with serious mental illnesses. We share your interest in improving care for this population, and others with mental illness, and look forward to continuing to work with you on this important issue.

As a Nation, we have come a long way in understanding the causes of serious mental illnesses and how to treat and support the people who experience them. Indeed, a snapshot of the mental health system in the 1950s would have shown a system that spent around 80 percent of its resources on warehousing people in institutions.[1] Modern day behavioral health care for those with the most serious illnesses offers new opportunities for rehabilitation and integration into society that would not have been conceivable half a

* This is an edited, reformatted and augmented version of testimony presented February 11, 2015 before the House Committee on Energy and Commerce, Subcommittee on Oversight and Investigations.

century ago. For example, during the 1950s and 1960s about 27 percent of people with serious mental illnesses were institutionalized and today it is only about seven percent (including those that are incarcerated).[2] Moreover, for people with serious mental illnesses, rates of treatment have grown dramatically. For example between 1990 and 2003 the percentage of people with serious mental illness receiving care increased by about 67 percent.[3] Nonetheless, serious mental illnesses can be devastating for individuals and families and much work is needed to reduce the burden of these disorders. We continue to work to address homelessness associated with those with serious mental illness, people with mental illness housed in the criminal justice system, and other painful consequences of people going without treatment and services.

OVERVIEW

HHS delivers treatment and supports to people with serious mental illnesses through its major health and social service programs – programs that serve this population along with Americans impacted by a wide range of diseases and conditions – as well as through specialized programs that provide targeted services to people with serious mental illness. HHS also conducts research on the biological processes that lead to serious mental illnesses. Although most of the funding for services for people with serious mental illnesses comes through our Federal insurance programs, especially Medicaid, the Substance Abuse and Mental Health Services Administration's (SAMHSA's) programs are critical in supporting the coordination of services for people with serious mental illnesses and improving the quality and accessibility of these services and supports. We agree with the U.S. Government Accountability Office (GAO) that coordination is essential for improving care and outcomes for people with serious mental illnesses, who have such complex health care and support needs. Thus, we work at many levels – inter-Departmental, inter-agency, and most importantly at the individual patient-level – to ensure the efficient and effective coordination of the programs and resources aimed at meeting those needs. Finally, we want to assure you of our commitment to program evaluation and accountability through performance measurement and that the Department and its agency components are working together to continuously improve our programs.

HOW WE CARE FOR PEOPLE WITH SERIOUS MENTAL ILLNESSES

Medicare, Medicaid, Supplemental Security Income, and Social Security Disability Insurance (SSDI) represent the largest sources of support for people with serious mental illnesses. With respect to mental health services, Medicaid and Medicare account for 40 percent of total spending on mental health care and a substantially larger portion of spending for people with serious mental disorders.[4] In fact, Medicaid is the single largest source of financing for mental health care in the United States including for people with serious mental illnesses (27 percent in 2009).[5] Federal funding for mental health services from all other sources accounts for five percent of total spending on mental health. The GAO report is focused on programs that make up this five percent of overall spending. While these programs, including the programs funded by SAMHSA, are important for development and implementation of evidence-based treatments, improving coordination of available resources and supports, broadening specialty care capacity and infrastructure, and collecting impact and general surveillance data, they make up a relatively small portion of HHS's overall spending on serious mental illnesses.

We expect millions of additional low-income adults with mental illness to gain coverage through the Medicaid expansion in the Affordable Care Act.[6] Recently, experts have estimated that Medicaid coverage expansion will also increase coverage for people with serious mental illnesses.[7] There is encouraging evidence from a pre-Affordable-Care-Act Oregon Medicaid demonstration that randomly assigned eligible individuals to a modest size Medicaid expansion. The evaluation of that effort showed, among other improved outcomes, increased care for depression resulting in lower levels of symptoms of depression in the newly covered population.[8] Improving access to mental health treatment through broad-based health and human service programs is a critical step toward improving outcomes for people with serious mental illness, who often are disengaged and disenfranchised as a result of their illness.[9]

Also not addressed in the GAO report is the increasingly important role that private health insurance plays in serving people with mental disorders,[10] particularly after enactment of the Mental Health Parity and Addiction Equity Act (MHPAEA) and the coverage expansions and protections for people with preexisting conditions in the Affordable Care Act. The Affordable Care Act also significantly extends the reach of the MHPAEA's requirements. The

Affordable Care Act requires all nongrandfathered small group and individual market plans to comply with Federal parity requirements. Qualified Health Plans offered through the Health Insurance Marketplace in every state must include coverage for mental and/or substance use disorders as one of the 10 categories of Essential Health Benefits, and that coverage must comply with the Federal parity requirements set forth in the MHPAEA. Emerging evidence, such as significant increases in health care coverage among young adults,[11] and dramatic upticks in utilization of inpatient care for mental health and substance use conditions in that population,[12] suggests that these reforms are improving access to mental health care. Similarly, recent findings from SAMHSA's National Survey on Drug Use and Health (NSDUH) show this expanded coverage has resulted in a significant rise in the percentage of young adults receiving mental health services in the past year – from 10.9 percent in 2010 to 11.9 percent in 2012. The study also shows that people in this age group who were insured were nearly twice as likely to receive mental health treatment as those without health insurance (13.5 percent versus 6.7 percent).

Targeted Programs Are Vital

The inclusion of mental health care into broader healthcare programs does not diminish the importance of targeted programs that direct specialized resources and expertise towards addressing the needs of people with serious mental illnesses and help us learn more about what works for them. Our success depends on making investments in specialized infrastructure and continuing our efforts to develop specialized treatment and support interventions. SAMHSA is central to this effort. The vast majority of SAMHSA's mental health spending targets individuals with serious mental illnesses. In FY 2014, over three-quarters of funding appropriated to SAMHSA for mental health services supported adults with or at risk for serious mental illnesses and/or children with serious emotional disturbances. This includes major programs such as the Community Mental Health Services Block Grant; the Children's Mental Health Initiative; and the Primary and Behavioral Health Care Integration (PBHCI) program. In addition, SAMHSA's homeless services programs, the largest of which are required in authorizing legislation to serve only those with serious mental illnesses, are prioritizing Veterans and people that are chronically homeless because such a high proportion of them have serious substance use disorders and/or serious mental issues.

The National Institute of Mental Health (NIMH) is also focused on improving care for individuals with serious mental illnesses through significant research investments to strengthen the evidence base for program and service delivery. One important project at NIMH is the Recovery After an Initial Schizophrenia Episode (RAISE) study. This study is a randomized controlled trial of specialized, team-based care for first episode psychosis in over 400 individuals at 34 community treatment centers across the United States. This project seeks to fundamentally change the trajectory and prognosis of schizophrenia through coordinated and aggressive treatment in the earliest stages of illness. Improving access to comprehensive specialized care is critically important to lessening the impact of serious mental illness. However, we know that, currently, it often takes over a year after a person first experiences psychosis – before they receive treatment for that condition.[13] As discussed in more detail below SAMHSA has been closely coordinating with NIMH to incorporate evidence developed from the RAISE project into SAMHSA's technical assistance efforts. Moving beyond first episode psychosis to earlier stages of psychosis risk, NIMH also developed the Early Psychosis Prediction and Prevention program to support high-quality research aimed at preventing psychosis onset among persons at clinical high-risk. NIMH funded five grants in FY 2014 that will inform a step-wise approach to clinical high-risk care that can be implemented rapidly in the U.S. healthcare system.

COORDINATION

There has been a long-standing interest among government officials and other stakeholders in improving coordination of the array of services and supports needed by people with serious mental illness.[14] Coordination can and should occur on multiple levels within the government and through a variety of means. Coordination can be achieved through formal interagency mechanisms, through program-level collaboration, or around a particular consumer's needs. We believe that coordination is needed at all levels, and a focus on consumer-centered care is critically important if outcomes are to improve for this very vulnerable population.

Consumer-Centered Care Coordination

People do not lead their lives according to program boundaries, and we have learned that we cannot run programs as if they do. That is why we devote substantial resources to models, programs, and demonstrations that focus on coordinating services for individuals across programs and agency boundaries. SAMHSA leads a number of our most important initiatives to coordinate services at the level of the individual beneficiary.

SAMHSA's Primary and Behavioral Health Care Integration (PBHCI) program is a prime example of how HHS' programs coordinate care for individual consumers through multi-agency cooperation. To date, over 125 community behavioral health centers across the United States have received PBHCI grants to provide integrated behavioral health and primary care services for adults with serious mental illnesses. Four main activities are required of PBHCI grantees: screening and referral for health care, systematically tracking consumers' physical health status and care needs, care management, and prevention and wellness services.

SAMHSA has worked with the Office of the Assistant Secretary for Planning and Evaluation (ASPE) at HHS on an evaluation of this program that found that the program increased access to primary care services, as well as improved health outcomes for individuals with serious mental illness with co-occurring diabetes, high cholesterol, and hypertension. As part of PBHCI, SAMHSA and the Health Resources and Services Administration (HRSA) co-fund the Center for Integrated Health Solutions (CIHS). CIHS promotes the development of integrated primary and behavioral health services to better address the needs of individuals with mental health and substance use conditions – especially those with serious mental illness, whether seen in behavioral-health or primary-care provider settings.

We also know that people with serious mental illnesses and their families often find themselves facing crisis situations in which the only available care is overworked emergency rooms often ill-equipped to address the needs of such individuals. That is why the President's FY 2016 Budget includes a new demonstration program in SAMHSA designed to help states and communities test the best way to structure, fund and deliver services to prevent, de-escalate and follow-up after behavioral health-related crises to assure the individual, family, community and delivery systems are adequately supported in such circumstances. The goal of this program is to test how best to reduce the need for inpatient care by providing earlier and more effective crisis services that bring multiple local, state and Federal funding sources together to adequately fund coordination of care across multiple settings and multiple community systems.

We also have a number of important care coordination initiatives focused on individuals with serious mental illnesses in HHS's broad-based programs. The health home option in Medicaid is focused on promoting care coordination for high-need individuals with an emphasis on people with serious mental illness. The health home benefit provides an enhanced Federal Medicaid match for care coordination, transitional care, linkages to community and social support services, and health information technology for individuals with multiple chronic conditions or a serious mental illness. Eligible providers include community mental health centers that are lynchpins of the public mental health care system. A number of states are targeting their health home benefits to individuals with serious mental illnesses, including New York, North Carolina, South Dakota, Vermont, Ohio and Missouri. In implementing the health home benefit, the Centers for Medicare & Medicaid Services (CMS) has collaborated closely with other agencies in the Department including SAMHSA and ASPE. For example, SAMHSA has helped review states' plans for health homes and provided consultation to states that focus this coordination benefit on individuals with mental illness or substance abuse. ASPE has been working with CMS to carry-out a five year evaluation of the health home option that will include detailed information on how states have implemented the benefit, as well as impacts on quality of care, inpatient and emergency room utilization, and costs for the individuals receiving this enhanced coordination benefit.

Our coordination efforts are especially evident with regard to the Department's work to improve coordination of care for those eligible for both Medicare and Medicaid, the "dual eligibles." We know that a high percentage of dual-eligible beneficiaries have serious mental health conditions.[15] These beneficiaries are among the sickest and poorest people covered by either Medicare or Medicaid. Integrated care demonstrations to coordinate service delivery and financing of both Medicare and Medicaid through a Federal-state collaboration have been implemented in twelve states.[16] The Massachusetts demonstration, for example, focuses on nonelderly dually eligible beneficiaries, a subpopulation of dually eligible beneficiaries with a high prevalence of serious mental illnesses and other behavioral health conditions. The Massachusetts demonstration incorporates an array of benefits designed to support persons with serious mental illness, including assertive community treatment, community crisis stabilization, psychiatric day treatment, and emergency services.

There are a number of new initiatives within Medicare focused on improving care coordination and promoting Accountable Care Organizations (ACOs), including the Medicare Shared Savings Program and the Pioneer ACO Model. Providers in these ACOs can receive shared savings for improving quality, care coordination, and reducing costs or pay shared losses in some cases for failing to meet certain benchmarks on quality and cost. These ACOs are accountable for care to Medicare beneficiaries assigned to the ACO, including individuals with serious mental illness.

SAMHSA also continues to prioritize and implement major programs designed to meet the needs of people with serious mental illness who experience criminal justice involvement, homelessness, and poverty (*e.g.*, Behavioral Health Treatment Court Collaborative, Cooperative Agreements to Benefit Homeless Individuals, and Projects for Assistance in Transition from Homelessness). For example, to improve consumer-centered coordination on the ground, SAMHSA administers the Cooperative Agreements to Benefit Homeless Individuals Program. The major goal of this program is to ensure, through state and local planning and service delivery, that Veterans who experience homelessness, as well as other homeless individuals (which is a population with high levels of serious mental illness), receive access to sustainable permanent housing, treatment, recovery supports, Medicaid and other benefits. Other SAMHSA programs that focus on care coordination for individuals with serious mental illness include the Behavioral Health Treatment Court Collaborative and Projects for Assistance in Transition from Homelessness.

Recently, SAMHSA has been working closely with CMS and ASPE to improve the quality and coordination of care for people with serious mental illness through implementation of a new demonstration program for Certified Community Behavioral Health Clinics established by the Protecting Access to Medicare Act. This program will provide enhanced Medicaid reimbursement for care coordination and comprehensive services at treatment centers that typically serve mostly individuals with serious mental illness. Just last week, SAMHSA released for public comment the draft criteria for community behavioral health clinics to be certified by states under the Section 223 demonstration program.

Participating centers will be required to meet staffing requirements, a comprehensive scope of services, standards for availability and accessibility of services, including prompt evaluation and crisis management services, and extensive requirements for enhanced care coordination. In addition, treatment centers will be required to report on quality measures that will include measures of care coordination. These data will inform an evaluation of this program that will be conducted by ASPE in close collaboration with SAMHSA and CMS.

Intra-Departmental Coordination

Beyond our focus on making sure services are coordinated for people with serious mental illness at the point of service, we are also engaged in efforts to coordinate across agencies within HHS. While the GAO report does not focus on coordination at the program level, we believe this is vital. Collaboration and coordination among programs can be very effective at ensuring Federal efforts are not inconsistent or overlapping. This collaboration at the program level is critical for ensuring that our best understanding of how to improve care for individuals with serious mental illness is being shared and implemented.

Established in 2010 by HHS, the Behavioral Health Coordinating Council's (BHCC) chief goals are to share information and ensure that all behavioral health issues are being handled collaboratively and without duplication of effort across the department. The BHCC's Serious Mental Illness Subcommittee is co-chaired by SAMHSA's Administrator and NIMH's Director and is helping to facilitate cross-agency collaborations. Topics that are a current focus of this subcommittee include: surveillance; early identification and intervention; engagement/outreach with consumers and their families such as psycho-education, peer and family support, shared decision-making, privacy and access to information issues; crisis response; provider capacity and training; and research priorities and opportunities for further collaboration across the Federal Government.

In addition to the cross-agency collaborations mentioned previously regarding PBHCI, Health Homes, and various other programs, SAMHSA has been closely coordinating with NIMH to incorporate information from the RAISE project into technical assistance for the states to use in implementing a new set-aside of Mental Health Block Grant funds for early intervention services. Recognizing the importance of engaging individuals with serious mental illnesses as early as possible in specialized services, the Congress recently required states to use five percent of the FY 2014 and FY 2015 Mental Health Block Grant funds they receive from SAMHSA to develop and support early intervention programs.[17] Multiple HHS agencies – including ASPE, SAMHSA, and NIMH – are working together to study how states are implementing the set-aside while also planning on a fuller evaluation of the impact of the set-aside in years to come.

Additionally, since 1989, SAMHSA has provided leadership by jointly funding, with the National Institute on Disability and Rehabilitation Research (NIDRR) of the Department of Education,[18] Research and Rehabilitation Training Centers that have conducted research on service delivery, employment, community living, health, and transition to adulthood for individuals with serious mental illness or serious emotional disturbance across their lifespan.

Inter-Departmental Coordination

At the interdepartmental level, there are also a number of coordinating bodies that focus on the needs of individuals with serious mental illness. Our approach to coordinating housing and services for the chronically homeless is an example of on the ground program coordination that is an outgrowth of Federal agencies reaching across program boundaries. The U.S. Interagency Council on Homelessness, co-chaired by Secretary Burwell along with Secretary Perez of the Department of Labor (DOL), has been invaluable in bringing together the resources and programs necessary to address the needs of individuals with chronic homelessness – the vast majority of whom have serious mental illness.

We also engage in direct collaborative work with other Departments including collaborations with the Department of Housing and Urban Development and the Social Security Administration (SSA) on efforts to coordinate care and support of people with serious mental illnesses. For instance, HHS has been engaged in a workgroup led by the Office of Management and Budget (OMB) that includes representatives from DOL, the Department of Education (ED), and SSA to develop a demonstration project for intervening earlier and diverting individuals from reliance on SSDI. We are now working across these departments to plan this demonstration that will primarily focus on people in the early stages of a serious mental illness. The intervention is in its early stages of development but will combine evidence based clinical care with well tested work support approaches.

In addition, SAMHSA leads both the Federal Working Group on Suicide Prevention and the Federal Partners Committee on Women and Trauma. The Administrator of SAMHSA also represents the HHS Secretary as co-chair of the Interagency Task Force on Military and Veterans Mental Health that includes HHS, ED, the Departments of Defense (DoD) and Veterans Affairs (VA), OMB, and the White House to address these and other issues affecting service members, Veterans and their families. Further efforts that exemplify SAMHSA's interagency coordination include the National Suicide Prevention Lifeline which SAMHSA co-leads with the VA, and the SAMHSA-funded National Action for Suicide Prevention, co-led by the Under Secretary of Defense for Personnel and Readiness, at DoD.

For people with serious mental illness, employment contributes to stability and independence. Unfortunately, many people with serious mental illness are unemployed. In FY 2014, SAMHSA initiated a new program, Transforming Lives through Supported Employment, to promote the employment of people with serious mental illness, and this initiative includes collaboration with ED, DOL, and states, among others.

We know that part of the answer to keeping individuals and their families supported and gainfully participating in regular community life is coordination across systems of care. Across many Departments, we have made significant investments in coordination because we know that it is one of the critical engines driving our programs to success.

We believe that our current methods of program coordination are robust and effective; however, we continue to look for ways to improve that coordination. As such, we take seriously GAO's recommendation to develop a more formal mechanism to further facilitate interagency coordination and thus enhance current coordination efforts.

Meaningful Program Evaluation is Key to Improving Services

GAO also challenges us to be rigorous about evaluation and performance measurement so we can monitor outcomes and progress. HHS is committed to evaluation of our programs, use of evaluation results in program design, and an ongoing process to improve the reach and quality of our evaluation efforts. ASPE is engaged in reviews of our approaches to evaluation across the Department. Our programs that serve people with serious mental illnesses are the subject of rigorous and ongoing evaluation to measure their impacts.

SAMHSA's Center for Behavioral Health Statistics and Quality includes a Quality, Evaluation, and Performance Branch which conducts a variety of evaluations of SAMHSA programs. A cross-agency SAMHSA Evaluation

Team helps determine which programs will be monitored through performance data and which programs will be evaluated more intensely through SAMHSA or external evaluation efforts. This branch also collaborates with ASPE, other HHS officials, and academic experts in planning, conducting, and reporting evaluation results to health professionals and the public. But SAMHSA's portfolio on evaluation work, like its investments in mental health system and service supports, is but one component of a multi-faceted evaluation approach.

Evaluations offer opportunities to coordinate across agencies regarding programs targeting individuals with serious mental illness. For example, ASPE has worked closely with SAMHSA for a number of years on an evaluation of the PBHCI program. In addition, ASPE is coordinating with CMS on an evaluation of the Medicaid health home benefit. Most recently, ASPE, SAMHSA, and CMS have been working together to develop the evaluation for the Certified Community Behavioral Health Clinic Demonstration. ASPE is also working with NIMH and SAMHSA to examine implementation of the set-aside of Mental Health Block Grant funds for early intervention services for individuals in the early stages of serious mental illness, including psychotic disorders.

ASPE, SAMHSA, and CMS are working together to look for opportunities to enhance the evaluation of HHS programs and also improve the availability of performance measures for monitoring the impact of our programs on people with serious mental illness Key to the success of evaluation is having strong performance measures. SAMHSA, working with ASPE, has funded the development and testing of a number of health care quality measures specific to people with serious mental illness. This work focuses on testing whether evidence-based care is being provided to persons with these conditions. Eleven of these measures have been submitted to and favorably reviewed by the National Quality Forum for measure endorsement as health plan quality measures. Such measures are part of SAMHSA's National Behavioral Health Quality Framework. NIMH and ASPE have also been co-leading an effort to develop a quality measure for evidence-based treatment for post-traumatic stress disorder. In addition, ASPE has been working with CMS to develop measures to include in the new reporting requirements in Medicare for inpatient psychiatric facilities – including a measure of whether individuals with serious mental illnesses coming out of these facilities are being adequately connected with services in the community.

In addition, NIMH, SAMHSA, VA, ASPE, and a number of mental health stakeholder groups have joined to fund the Institute of Medicine to chart a course forward on improving the quality of psychosocial interventions.

LESSONS LEARNED

While we look for opportunities to continuously update and improve our programs, we have learned a lot about what works and what needs to be emphasized in supporting people with serious mental illness.

First and foremost, services must be coordinated on the ground so that they meet the often complex needs of people with serious mental illnesses. This is especially the case when the vast majority of services and supports for people with these conditions are delivered through general health and income support programs.

Second, coordination at high levels of Government is desirable and can help meet the needs of people at the point of service.

Third, coordination at the level of agencies that directly interact with people receiving publicly or privately funded services is vitally important.

Coordination at each of these levels is needed to best serve the needs of individuals with serious mental illness – and we are committed to achieving that goal.

Much progress has been made over the past half century and there have been many champions along the way. We look forward to partnering with the Congress to continue to improve care for individuals with the most serious mental illnesses.

End Notes

[1] Frank RG, Glied SA. Better But Not Well: Mental Health Policy in the United States Since 1950. Baltimore: The Johns Hopkins University Press, 2006.

[2] Frank and Glied see note 1.

[3] Kessler RC et al, US Prevalence and Treatment of Mental Disorders 1990-2003; New England J Medicine 352 (24) 2515-2523, 2005.

[4] Substance Abuse and Mental Health Services Administration. National Expenditures for Mental Health Services and Substance Abuse Treatment, 1986–2009. HHS Publication No. SMA-13-4740. Rockville, MD: Substance Abuse and Mental Health Services Administration, 2013. Available on-line at http://store.samhsa.gov/product/National-Expenditures-for-Mental-Health-Services-and-Substance-AbuseTreatment-1986-2009/SMA13-4740.

[5] Id.

[6] Garfield RL, Zuvekas SH, Lave JR, et al. The Impact of National Health Care Reform on Adults with Severe Mental Disorders. American Journal of Psychiatry. 2011; 168(5): 486-494.

[7] Mark TL, Weir LM, Malone K, et al. National Estimates of Behavioral Health Conditions and their Treatment Among Adults Newly Insured under the Affordable Care Act. Psychiatric Services in Advance, accessed on-line February 3, 2015.

[8] Baicker K, Taubman SL, Allen HL, et al. The Oregon Experiment – Effects of Medicaid on Clinical Outcomes. N Engl J Med. 2013 May 2; 368(18): 1713-1722.

[9] See, e.g., American Mental Health Counselors Association, Broken Promises; More Despair; How the Lack of State Participation in the Medicaid Expansion Will Punish Americans with Mental Illness. February 2014. Available online at http://www.amhca.org/assets/content/AMHCA_DashedHopes_Report_2_21_14_final.pdf.

[10] Mark TL, Weir LM, Malone K, et al. National Estimates of Behavioral Health Conditions and their Treatment Among Adults Newly Insured under the Affordable Care Act. Psychiatric Services in Advance, accessed on-line February 3, 2015.

[11] Martinez ME, Cohen RA. Health Insurance Coverage: Early Release of Estimates from the National Health Interview Survey, January-September, 2012. March 2013. Available online at http://www.cdc.gov/nchs/data/nhis/earlyrelease/Insur201303.pdf.

[12] Health Care Cost Institute, Issue Brief No. 8: Selected Health Care Trends for Young Adults (ages 19025): 2007- 2012. September 2014. Available online at www. healthco stinstitute.org.

[13] Addington J, Heinssen RK, Robinson DG, et al. Duration of Untreated Psychosis in Community Treatment Settings in the United States. Psychiatric Services in Advance. Accessed on-line February 3, 2015.

[14] Frank RG, Glied SA. Better But Not Well: Mental Health Policy in the United States Since 1950. Baltimore: The Johns Hopkins University Press, 2006.

[15] Medicare Payment Advisory Commission and Medicaid and CHIP Payment and Access Commission. Data Book: Beneficiaries Dually Eligible for Medicare and Medicaid. January 2015. Available on-line at http://www.macpac.gov/publications; Frank RG, Epstein AM. Factors Associated with High Levels of Spending for Younger Dually Eligible Beneficiaries with Mental Disorders. Health Affairs. June 2014; 33(6): 1006-1013.

[16] CA, CO, IL, MA, MI, MN, NY, OH, SC, TX, VA, and WA.

[17] Approximately $24.2 million in funds each year.

[18] With the signing of the Workforce Innovation and Opportunity Act of 2014, NIDRR became the National Institute on Disability, Independent Living, and Rehabilitation Research, and was moved to the Administration for Community Living in HHS.

In: Federal Programs
Editor: Benjamin Wright

ISBN: 978-1-63483-043-0

Chapter 3

PREVALENCE OF MENTAL ILLNESS IN THE UNITED STATES: DATA SOURCES AND ESTIMATES*

Erin Bagalman and Angela Napili

SUMMARY

Determining how many people have a mental illness can be difficult, and prevalence estimates vary. While numerous surveys include questions related to mental illness, few provide prevalence estimates of *diagnosable mental illness* (e.g., major depressive disorder as opposed to feeling depressed, or generalized anxiety disorder as opposed to feeling anxious), and fewer still provide *national* prevalence estimates of diagnosable mental illness. This report briefly describes the methodology and results of three large surveys (funded in whole or in part by the U.S. Department of Health and Human Services) that provide *national prevalence estimates of diagnosable mental illness*: the National Comorbidity Survey Replication (NCS-R), the National Comorbidity Survey Replication Adolescent Supplement (NCS-A), and the National Survey on Drug Use and Health (NSDUH). The NCS-R and the NCS-A have the advantage of identifying specific mental illnesses, but they are

* This is an edited, reformatted and augmented version of a Congressional Research Service publication R43047, prepared for Members and Committees of Congress, dated March 9, 2015.

more than a decade old. The NSDUH does not identify specific mental illnesses, but it has the advantage of being conducted annually.

Between February 2001 and April 2003, NCS-R staff interviewed more than 9,000 adults aged 18 or older. Analyses of NCS-R data have yielded different prevalence estimates. One analysis of NCS-R data estimated that 26.2% of adults had a mental illness within a 12-month period (hereinafter called 12-month prevalence). Another analysis of NCS-R data estimated the 12-month prevalence of mental illness to be 32.4% among adults. A third analysis of NCS-R data estimated the 12-month prevalence of mental illness *excluding substance use disorders* to be 24.8% among adults. The 12-month prevalence of *serious* mental illness was estimated to be 5.8% among adults, based on NCS-R data.

Between February 2001 and January 2004, NCS-A staff interviewed more than 10,000 adolescents aged 13 to 17. Using NCS-A data, researchers estimated the 12-month prevalence of mental illness to be 40.3% among adolescents. Some have suggested that the current approach to diagnosing mental illness identifies people who should not be considered mentally ill. The 12- month prevalence of *serious* mental illness was estimated to be 8.0% among adolescents, based on NCS-A data.

The NSDUH is an annual survey of approximately 70,000 adults and adolescents aged 12 years or older in the United States. According to the 2013 NSDUH, the estimated 12-month prevalence of mental illness *excluding substance use disorders* was 18.5% among adults aged 18 or older. The estimated 12-month prevalence of *serious* mental illness (excluding substance use disorders) was 4.2% among adults. Although the NSDUH collects information related to mental illness (e.g., symptoms of depression) from adolescents aged 12 to 17, it does not produce estimates of mental illness for that population.

The prevalence estimates discussed in this report may raise questions for Congress. Should federal mental health policy focus on adults or adolescents with *any* mental illness (including some whose mental illnesses may be mild and even transient) or on those with *serious* mental illness? Should substance use disorders be addressed through the same policies as other mental illnesses? Members of Congress may approach mental health policy differently depending in part on how they answer such questions.

INTRODUCTION

Congress has demonstrated an interest in mental health and mental illness,[1] and knowing how many people have a mental illness may be helpful in addressing related policy issues. Determining how many people have a mental illness can be difficult, and prevalence[2] estimates vary. While numerous surveys include questions related to mental illness, few provide prevalence estimates of *diagnosable mental illness*, and fewer still provide *national* prevalence estimates of diagnosable mental illness.[3]

This report briefly describes the methodology and selected findings of three large federally funded surveys that provide *national prevalence estimates of diagnosable mental illness*: the National Comorbidity Survey Replication (NCS-R), the National Comorbidity Survey Replication Adolescent Supplement (NCS-A), and the National Survey on Drug Use and Health (NSDUH). This report presents prevalence estimates of *any* mental illness and *serious* mental illness[4] based on each survey and ends with a brief discussion of how these prevalence estimates might inform policy discussions.

One data source may be preferred over another in specific situations. For example, the NCS-R and the NCS-A are more than a decade old, so the NSDUH (which is conducted annually) may be preferred for more recent prevalence estimates. On the other hand, the NCS-R and the NCS-A provide prevalence estimates for specific disorders,[5] which the NSDUH does not provide.[6]

ESTIMATING PREVALENCE OF MENTAL ILLNESS

In clinical practice, mental health professionals diagnose mental illnesses based on criteria in the American Psychiatric Association's *Diagnostic and Statistical Manual of Mental Disorders* (DSM)[7] and exercise clinical judgment in doing so.[8] Large surveys, however, may not allow for lengthy interviews and use of clinical judgment. Considerations in generating national prevalence estimates of diagnosable mental illness[9] through large surveys include (1) what survey instrument (i.e., set of questions) is used, (2) who administers it, and (3) how generalizable the findings are. Each of these considerations is discussed briefly below.

When designing surveys, researchers must weigh the value of detailed information against the time required to collect that information. Longer survey instruments may be better able to identify mental illness accurately by asking all or most of the questions necessary to assess DSM diagnostic criteria. Shorter survey instruments, while more practical to include in a survey, may not identify mental illness as accurately as longer instruments. *Table 1* provides examples of survey instruments assessing mental illness.

Survey instruments may be administered in different ways, which may affect both the accuracy of their assessment of mental illness and the feasibility of their inclusion in large surveys. Some, such as the Structured Clinical Interview for DSM Disorders (described in *Table 1*), require trained mental health professionals. Others require trained interviewers who need not be mental health professionals. Still others may be self-administered or administered by interviewers without extensive training.

The prevalence estimates described in this report are weighted to reflect the general U.S. population as closely as possible.[10] This is accomplished by assigning a weight to each survey respondent based on information that is available for both the survey respondents and the general U.S. population (e.g., age and gender, among others). Weighting can correct for known differences between the survey respondents and the general U.S. population (e.g., if people in a certain age range are overrepresented in the survey). Weighting cannot, however, correct for subpopulations that are excluded from the survey altogether (e.g., the homeless). Prevalence estimates are not generalizable to excluded subpopulations.[11]

Table 1. Examples of Survey Instruments Assessing Mental Illness

Instrument	What It Assesses	Who Administers It	How Long It Takes	Examples of Surveys Using It
Structured Clinical Interview for DSM Disorders (SCID)[a]	Diagnoses	Trained mental health professionals	Approximately 30–60 minutes	NSDUH (for a subsample of respondents)
World Mental Health Survey Initiative version of the Composite International Diagnostic Interview (WMH-CIDI)[b]	Diagnoses, functioning, treatment, risk factors, socio-demographic characteristics, and more	Trained lay interviewers	Approximately 2 hours, but modular so that some sections can be excluded	NCS-R; NCS-A uses a modified Composite International Diagnostic Interview (CIDI)
World Health Organization Disability Assessment Schedule (WHODAS)[c]	Difficulties (due to health conditions) in the areas of cognition, mobility, self-care, getting along, life activities, and participation	Either self-administered or administered by an interviewer (no training required)	Different versions are available; the longest (36 items) takes approximately 15–20 minutes	NSDUH uses a modified version

Instrument	What It Assesses	Who Administers It	How Long It Takes	Examples of Surveys Using It
Kessler-6 Psychological Distress Scale (K6)[d]	Frequency and severity of feeling nervous, hopeless, restless/fidgety, sad/depressed, and worthless	Either self-administered or administered by an interviewer (no training required)	No more than 2 minutes	NSDUH uses a modified version

Note: A survey instrument is a tool for systematically collecting information from survey respondents; each instrument listed in this table is a set of questions that may be asked as part of a larger questionnaire.

[a] DSM = Diagnostic and Statistical Manual of Mental Disorders. Information about the SCID in this table is drawn from U.S. Department of Health and Human Services (HHS), Centers for Disease Control and Prevention (CDC), "Mental Illness Surveillance in the United States," Morbidity and Mortality Weekly Report, vol. 60, Supplement (September 2, 2011).

[b] Information about the WMH-CIDI in this table is drawn from Ronald C. Kessler and T. Bedirhan Üstün, "The World Mental Health (WMH) Survey Initiative Version of the World Health Organization (WHO) Composite International Diagnostic Interview (CIDI)," International Journal of Methods in Psychiatric Research, vol. 13, no. 2 (2004), pp. 93-121.

[c] Information about the WHODAS in this table is drawn from World Health Organization, Classifications, Classification of Functioning, Disability and Health (ICF), http://www.who.int/classifications/icf/whodasii/en/.

[d] Ronald C. Kessler et al., "Screening for Serious Mental Illness in the General Population with the K6 Screening Scale: Results from the WHO World Mental Health (WMH) Survey Initiative," International Journal of Methods in Psychiatric Research, vol. 19 (Supplement 1) (2010), pp. 4-22.

National Comorbidity Survey Replication

The National Comorbidity Survey Replication (NCS-R) replicated the original National Comorbidity Survey (conducted between 1990 and 1992), which was the first survey to use fully structured research diagnostic interviews to assess a wide range of DSM disorders among a national sample of adults in the United States.[12] The NCS-R was funded primarily by the National Institute of Mental Health within the National Institutes of Health (NIH) of the Department of Health and Human Services (HHS), with supplemental support from the National Institute on Drug Abuse (also within NIH), the Substance Abuse and Mental Health Services Administration (of HHS), the Robert Wood Johnson Foundation, and the John W. Alden Trust.[13]

Between February 2001 and April 2003, NCS-R staff conducted in-person interviews with more than 9,000 adults aged 18 or older, drawing the sample from households in the contiguous United States. The sample did not include the homeless, individuals in institutions, or non-English speakers; these exclusions limit the generalizability of findings based on the NCS-R.[14]

Prevalence of Any Mental Illness Among Adults

The NCS-R determined the presence of any mental illness based on the World Health Organization's World Mental Health Survey Initiative version of the Composite International Diagnostic Interview (WMH-CIDI), which assessed 19 specific DSM diagnoses.[15] Analyses of NCS-R data have yielded different prevalence estimates. One analysis of NCS-R data estimated that 26.2% of adults had a mental illness within a 12-month period (hereinafter called 12-month prevalence).[16] Another analysis of NCS-R data estimated the 12-month prevalence of mental illness to be 32.4% among adults; the difference may be attributable to the use of more recent information about the U.S. population in weighting the NCS-R data.[17] Both of these estimates include substance use disorders as mental illness; an analysis of NCS-R data estimated the 12- month prevalence of mental illness *excluding substance use disorders* to be 24.8% among adults.[18]

Prevalence of Serious Mental Illness Among Adults

Additional analyses of NSC-R data were conducted to determine the 12-month prevalence of mental illness at three levels of severity: serious,[19] moderate,[20] or mild.[21] Among the 26.2% of adults identified with a mental disorder in the analysis, serious disorders (22.3% *among adults with a disorder*) were less common than moderate disorders (37.3%) or mild disorders (40.4%). The estimated 12-month prevalence of serious mental illness among *all* adults was 5.8%.[22]

National Comorbidity Survey Replication Adolescent Supplement

The National Comorbidity Survey Replication Adolescent Supplement (NCS-A) was the first survey to use fully structured research diagnostic interviews to assess a wide range of DSM disorders among a national sample of adolescents in the United States. Like the NCS-R, the NCSA was funded primarily by the National Institute of Mental Health, with supplemental support from the National Institute on Drug Abuse, the Substance Abuse and Mental Health Services Administration, the Robert Wood Johnson Foundation, and the John W. Alden Trust.[23] Between February 2001 and January 2004, NCS-A staff interviewed more than 10,000 adolescents aged 13 to 17, drawing the sample from both schools and households in the coterminous United States. Adolescent participants were interviewed in person, and one parent of each participating adolescent was asked to complete a self-administered questionnaire about the adolescent's developmental history and mental health. The sample did not include the homeless, individuals in institutions, or non-English speakers; these exclusions limit the generalizability of findings based on the NCS-A.[24]

Prevalence of Any Mental Illness Among Adolescents

The NCS-A determined the presence of any mental illness based on a modified Composite International Diagnostic Interview (CIDI), which assessed 15 specific DSM diagnoses. Using NCS-A data, researchers estimated the 12-month prevalence of mental illness to be 40.3% among adolescents.[25] Some have suggested that the current version of the DSM identifies people who should not be considered mentally ill.[26]

Prevalence of Serious Mental Illness Among Adolescents

Additional analyses of NCS-A data were conducted to determine the presence of serious mental illness (called serious emotional disturbance in NCS-A), which was defined as at least one diagnosis accompanied by an estimated score of 50 or less on the Children's Global Assessment Scale (CGAS), indicating either severe functional impairment in one area of living or moderate functional impairment in most areas of living. The CGAS score was not measured directly as part of the NCS-A. Instead the NCS-A used a sophisticated approach that involved (1) selection of a subsample of 347 adolescent-parent pairs from the main study; (2) follow-up telephone interviews conducted by mental health professionals who assigned CGAS scores; (3) development of a statistical model linking CGAS scores to responses to questions in the main study; and (4) application of the statistical model to the full sample to impute CGAS scores based on responses to questions in the main study.[27]

Using the imputed CGAS scores, researchers assessed serious mental illness among 6,483 adolescent NCS-A participants with complete data (including parent questionnaires). This analysis yielded a 12-month prevalence of any mental illness (42.6%) that was slightly higher than the previous estimate and found most cases to be mild (58.2% *among adolescents with a disorder*) or moderate (22.9%), rather than serious (18.8%). The estimated 12-month prevalence of serious mental illness among *all* adolescents was 8.0%. Some people have suggested that most adolescents with mental disorders do not need treatment because their disorders are mild and will resolve on their own; however, some research has shown that mild disorders during adolescence may predict serious disorders during adulthood.[28]

NATIONAL SURVEY ON DRUG USE AND HEALTH

The National Survey on Drug Use and Health (NSDUH) focuses primarily on the use of illegal drugs, alcohol, and tobacco and also includes several modules that focus on mental health issues.[29] The NSDUH is funded by the Substance Abuse and Mental Health Services Administration. Each year, the NSDUH surveys approximately 70,000 non-institutionalized civilians aged 12 years or older in the United States, divided roughly between 45,000 adults (aged 18 or older) and 25,000 adolescents (aged 12 to 17).[30] The NSDUH is conducted in both English and Spanish. Participants are interviewed in their homes using a combination of personal interviewing and audio computer-assisted self-interviewing, which offers more privacy in order to encourage honest reporting of sensitive topics such as illicit drug use. The sample does not include homeless persons not living in a shelter, individuals in institutions, those who speak a language other than English or Spanish, or military personnel on active duty; these exclusions limit the generalizability of findings based on the NSDUH.[31]

NSDUH-based prevalence estimates of any mental illness and serious mental illness among adults aged 18 or older are described below. Although the NSDUH collects information related to mental illness (e.g., symptoms of depression) from adolescents aged 12 to 17, it does not produce *prevalence estimates of mental illness* for that population.

Prevalence of Any Mental Illness Among Adults

The NSDUH determines the presence of any mental illness based on a combination of relatively short modules of questions (including modified versions of the K6 and WHODAS described in *Table 1*) in the main survey and information from an additional follow-up interview conducted with a subsample of adults from the main survey.[32] Unlike the NCS-R and the NCS-A, the core component of NSDUH does not include questions designed to identify specific DSM diagnoses. Instead, the NSDUH uses an approach similar to the one used by NCS-A to impute the CGAS, involving (1) selection of a subsample of adults from the main study; (2) follow-up telephone interviews conducted by mental health professionals who conduct the Structured Clinical Interview for DSM Disorders (SCID); (3) development of a statistical model linking the SCIDbased diagnosis of mental illness to responses to questions in the main study; and (4) application of the statistical model to the full sample to impute the presence of mental illness based on responses to questions in the main study.[33] According to the 2013 NSDUH, the estimated 12-month prevalence of mental illness *excluding substance use disorders* is 18.5% of adults (aged 18 or older).[34]

Prevalence of Serious Mental Illness Among Adults

The NSDUH identifies adults (aged 18 or older) as having a serious mental illness if (1) they have a mental illness (excluding substance use disorders and developmental disorders) and (2) the illness substantially interferes with or limits at least one major life activity. The same approach used to impute any mental illness is applied to impute serious mental illness. According to the 2013 NSDUH, the estimated 12-month prevalence of serious mental illness *excluding substance use disorders* is 4.2% among adults (aged 18 or older).[35]

CONCLUDING COMMENTS

Knowing how many people are likely to be affected by policies related to mental illness may help policy makers identify specific problems as well as their scope; however, the national prevalence estimates discussed in this report may raise as many questions as they answer. For example, given the difference in prevalence estimates between *any* mental illness and *serious* mental illness among adolescents, might policy makers choose to focus on a large group of adolescents that includes many whose mental illnesses may be mild and even transient, or might they choose to focus more narrowly on adolescents with serious mental illness? As clinical practice is moving toward more integrated care,[36] should substance use disorders be included in the definition of mental illness (as in the NCS-R and the NCS-A) and addressed through the same policies, or should they be identified separately (as in the NSDUH) and addressed through different policies? How might policy makers address mental illness among populations that are excluded from the prevalence estimates (e.g., the homeless)? With regard to the NCS-R and the NCS-A, there is an overarching question of whether prevalence estimates based on surveys conducted more than a decade ago remain relevant to current policy discussions. Policy makers may come to different conclusions about the best policy approach depending in part on how they answer such questions.

End Notes

[1] See, for example, U.S. Congress, Senate Committee on Health, Education, Labor, & Pensions, Examining Mental Health: Treatment Options and Trends, 113th Cong., 2nd sess., February 25, 2014, http://www.help.senate.gov/hearings/ hearing/?id=b7f1350d-5056-a032-5216-4bb68fe0bcee; and U.S. Congress, House Committee on Energy and Commerce, Subcommittee on Oversight and Investigations, Where Have All the Patients Gone? Examining the Psychiatric Bed Shortage 113th Cong., 2nd sess., March 26, 2014, http://purl.fdlp.gov/GPO/gpo52981.

[2] Prevalence is the share of a population affected by a given condition during a specified period of time. The term "12- month prevalence" refers to the share of study participants with symptoms that could be identified as mental illness in the 12 months before the interview. Another way to express prevalence is "lifetime prevalence," which is based on the share of study participants that had ever had a mental illness as of the time of the interview. This report focuses on 12- month prevalence because it more closely reflects the number of people with mental illness at a given time, which might translate into need for services at a given time.

[3] See U.S. Department of Health and Human Services (HHS), Centers for Disease Control and Prevention (CDC), "Mental Illness Surveillance in the United States," Morbidity and

Mortality Weekly Report, vol. 60, Supplement (September 2, 2011), http://www.cdc.gov/mmwr/preview/mmwrhtml/su6003a1.htm; and HHS, Substance Abuse and Mental Health Services Administration (SAMHSA), Center for Behavioral Health Statistics and Quality (CBHSQ), Comparison of NSDUH Mental Health Data and Methods with Other Data Sources, March 2012, http://www.samhsa.gov/data/NSDUH/2k12Findings/CBHSQDataReviewC2MentalHealth2012.pdf.

[4] Severity of mental illness is generally defined by the number of symptoms (i.e., whether the individual has just enough symptoms to meet diagnostic criteria or has excess symptoms) and/or the degree of functional impairment (e.g., whether an individual with mental illness is unable to work as a consequence of the illness). Each survey discussed in this report uses its own definition of serious mental illness.

[5] Estimates of specific disorders are not presented in this report; they are available in the cited documents.

[6] The NSDUH provides more detailed information about substance use disorders, but not other mental illness.

[7] American Psychiatric Association, Diagnostic and Statistical Manual of Mental Disorders, Fifth Edition (DSM-5), (Washington, DC: American Psychiatric Association, 2013). Some of the interviews designed for research are based on the fourth edition, text revision (DSM-IV-TR), published in 2000, or the fourth edition prior to the text revision (DSMIV), published in 1994.

[8] A diagnosis of mental illness may be based on what an individual reports about himself or herself; what other people report about the individual (if, for example, a family member is available); and what the mental health professional observes about the individual. People may not be forthcoming with information about certain behaviors (e.g., drug use) or symptoms (e.g., hallucinations); this is a challenge in both clinical settings and research settings.

[9] This report uses the term "diagnosable" as distinct from "diagnosed" in acknowledgement of the potential for surveys to identify people suffering from mental illnesses that have not been diagnosed by a mental health professional. Also important is the distinction between symptoms of mental illness (e.g., feelings of depression or anxiety) and a combination of symptoms meeting DSM criteria for a diagnosis of mental illness (e.g., major depressive disorder or generalized anxiety disorder). While all DSM disorders may be considered mental illnesses, surveys generally do not assess all of them. In this report, some of the prevalence estimates include substance use disorders and others do not.

[10] The weighting was done by the researchers whose published results CRS cites in this report, not by CRS.

[11] Excluded subpopulations may have higher or lower risk of mental illness than the general population. Thus if these subpopulations had been included in the surveys, the overall prevalence estimates would have been slightly higher or lower accordingly. Policy approaches that might be appropriate for excluded subpopulations such as the homeless or non-English speakers may be different than policy approaches for the general population.

[12] Harvard Medical School, Department of Health Care Policy, National Comorbidity Survey, http://www.hcp.med.harvard.edu/ncs/.

[13] Ronald C. Kessler et al., "Prevalence, Severity, and Comorbidity of Twelve-month DSM-IV Disorders in the National Comorbidity Survey Replication (NCS-R)," Archives of General Psychiatry, vol. 62, no. 6 (June 2005), pp. 617-627. Hereinafter, Kessler et al., NCS-R Prevalence, (2005).

[14] Kessler et al., NCS-R Prevalence, (2005).

[15] The DSM includes more than 19 diagnoses. While all of them may be considered mental illnesses, some are often excluded from definitions of mental illness (e.g., learning disorders).

[16] Kessler et al., NCS-R Prevalence, (2005).

[17] Harvard Medical School, Department of Health Care Policy, National Comorbidity Survey, "NSC-R Twelve-Month Prevalence Estimates" link at http://www.hcp.med. harvard. edu/ncs/. This later analysis was based on updated data as of July 19, 2007, and "reflect[s] the latest diagnostic, demographic and raw variable information."

[18] Benjamin G. Druss et al. "Impairment in Role Functioning in Mental and Chronic Medical Disorders in the United States: Results from the National Comorbidity Survey Replication." Molecular Psychiatry, vol. 14, no. 7 (July 2009), pp. 728-737.

[19] Kessler et al., NCS-R Prevalence, (2005). Any of the following qualified a case of mental illness as serious: "a 12- month suicide attempt with serious lethality intent; work disability or substantial limitation due to a mental or substance disorder; positive screen results for non-affective psychosis; bipolar I or II disorder; substance dependence with serious role impairment (as defined by disorder-specific impairment questions); an impulse control disorder with repeated serious violence; or any disorder that resulted in 30 or more days out of role in the year" (p. 618).

[20] Kessler et al., NCS-R Prevalence, (2005). Among cases of mental illness not defined as serious, any of the following qualified a case as moderate: "suicide gesture, plan, or ideation; substance dependence without serious role impairment; at least moderate work limitation due to a mental or substance disorder; or any disorder with at least moderate role impairment in 2 or more domains of the Sheehan Disability Scale [which] assessed disability in work role performance, household maintenance, social life, and intimate relationships" (p. 618).

[21] Kessler et al., NCS-R Prevalence, (2005). All cases of mental illness that were not defined as serious or moderate were considered mild (p. 618).

[22] Kessler et al., NCS-R Prevalence, (2005).

[23] Ronald C. Kessler et al., "Prevalence, Persistence, and Sociodemographic Correlates of DSM-IV Disorders in the National Comorbidity Survey Replication Adolescent Supplement," Archives of General Psychiatry, vol. 69, no. 4 (April 2012). Hereinafter, Kessler et al., NCS-A Prevalence, (2012).

[24] Ronald C. Kessler et al., "Severity of 12-Month DSM-IV Disorders in the National Comorbidity Survey Replication Adolescent Supplement," Archives of General Psychiatry, vol. 69, no. 4 (April 2012). Hereinafter, Kessler et al., NCSA Severity, (2012).

[25] Kessler et al., NCS-A Prevalence, (2012).

[26] Kessler et al., NCS-A Severity, (2012).

[27] Kessler et al., NCS-A Prevalence, (2012); Kessler et al., NCS-A Severity, (2012); and Ronald C. Kessler et al., "The National Comorbidity Survey Adolescent Supplement (NCSA): III. Concordance of DSM-IV/CIDI Diagnoses with Clinical Reassessments," Journal of the American Academy of Child and Adolescent Psychiatry, vol. 48, no. 4 (April 2009), pp. 386-399.

[28] Kessler et al., NCS-A Severity, (2012).

[29] U.S. Department of Health and Human Services (HHS), Substance Abuse and Mental Health Services Administration (SAMHSA), Center for Behavioral Health Statistics and Quality (CBHSQ), Substance Use and Mental Health Estimates from the 2013 National Survey on Drug Use and Health: Overview of Findings NSDUH14-0904, Rockville, MD, September

4, 2014, http://store.samhsa.gov/shin/content//NSDUH14-0904/NSDUH14-0904.pdf. Hereinafter, 2013 NSDUH: Overview of Findings.

[30] In 2013, 67,838 respondents completed a NSDUH interview, including 45,344 adults and 22,494 adolescents. (2013 NSDUH: Overview of Findings, p. 8).

[31] HHS, SAMHSA, Results from the 2013 National Survey on Drug Use and Health: Summary of National Findings, NSDUH Series H-48, HHS Publication No. (SMA) 14-4863, Rockville, MD, 2014, pp. 113, 129, http://www.samhsa.gov/data/sites/default/files/NSDUHresultsPDFWHTML2013/Web/NSDUHresults2013.pdf. Hereinafter, 2013 NSDUH: Summary of National Findings. The NSDUH has been ongoing since 1971; prior to 2002, it was called the National Household Survey on Drug Abuse.

[32] 2013 NSDUH: Summary of National Findings, pp. 115-117; HHS, SAMHSA, Results from the 2013 National Survey on Drug Use and Health: Mental Health Findings, NSDUH Series H-49, HHS Publication No. (SMA) 14-4887. Rockville, MD, 2014, http://www.samhsa.gov/data/sites/default/files/NSDUHmhfr2013/NSDUHmhfr2013.pdf. See Appendix B: Statistical Methods and Measurement, B.4.3 Estimation of Serious and Other Levels of Mental Illness.

[33] This approach, called the Mental Health Surveillance Study, began with the 2008 NSDUH. The statistical model was changed in 2012; the 2012 model continued to be used in 2013.

[34] 2013 NSDUH: Overview of Findings, p. 6.

[35] 2013 NSDUH: Overview of Findings, p. 6.

[36] Like clinical practice, financing is moving toward including substance use disorders with the rest of mental illness. The Mental Health Parity Act of 1996 (MHPA, P.L. 104-204) did not apply to coverage of substance use disorders. The more recent Paul Wellstone and Pete Domenici Mental Health Parity and Addiction Equity Act of 2008 (MHPAEA, P.L. 110-343) applies to both substance use disorders and the rest of mental illness.

INDEX

D

E

F

G

H

I

L

M

N

O

P

Q

R

S